SERVICE BEFORE SELF

Responding to the 2014–2016 Ebola Crisis

USPHS Commissioned Corps Health Services Officers

Service Before Self: Responding to the 2014–2016 Ebola Crisis

https://www.phscof.org/

Cover photo by Evan Schneider

Cover Photo Caption: *Health Services Officer LCDR Matthew Johns in personal protective equipment (PPE) at the Ebola Treatment Unit (ETU) in Monrovia, Liberia*

Editor's Note: *In the following pages, you will see photographs of USPHS Commissioned Corps officers not in uniform. Officers deploying under orders from the Commissioned Corps Readiness and Deployment Branch (formerly known as RedDOG) are seen in uniform. Officers deployed by their respective agencies may have specific agency requirements restricting them from deploying in uniform, depending on their mission and its location. Also, many of the officers have changed rank since the deployment; this work reflects their rank at the time of deployment. Quotes have been edited for repetition, clarity, and consistency.*

Cover Design: Deborah Bradseth at Tugboat Design, LLC

Editing: Amy M. Carlin

Interior Design & Layout: Melissa Williams Design

SERVICE BEFORE SELF

This collection of original stories is dedicated to all United States Public Health Service (USPHS) health services officers (HSOs) who bravely served on the frontlines during the international Ebola crisis between 2014 and 2016, in addition to the officers serving in integral mission operations and those who stepped up to continue critical agency assignments impacted by the deployments of the frontline responders.

Using the framework of the Global Health Security Agenda, this collection is organized into three distinct sections-Detect, Prevent, Respond. Here, officers share firsthand accounts of how they served as hope multipliers in a time of crisis. Because of the unprecedented nature of this response, leading to the most visible and widely recognized global health response in USPHS Commissioned Corps history, the HSO category wanted to memorialize these stories, which are also our USPHS Commissioned Corps stories.

Within these pages, we honor officers serving in the highest levels of leadership who were critically important to mission success. The history brought to life here demonstrates the HSO motto "Multidisciplinary in approach, connected by service, advancing public health," attesting to the wide range of skills and experience possessed by these officers, which was brought to bear on the 2014–2016 Ebola response.

A tremendous debt of gratitude is owed to the federal agencies and tribal organizations who supported officers with salaries and time away from their duty stations while they were deployed for up to four months. The USPHS Commissioned Corps and, equally—the Health Services category—stand ready to respond in future times of crisis and public health need, which are sure to come in an ever-changing world.

"The deployment was something that most people work their entire career to be part of."

—Matthew Johns, MPH, LCDR, USPHS

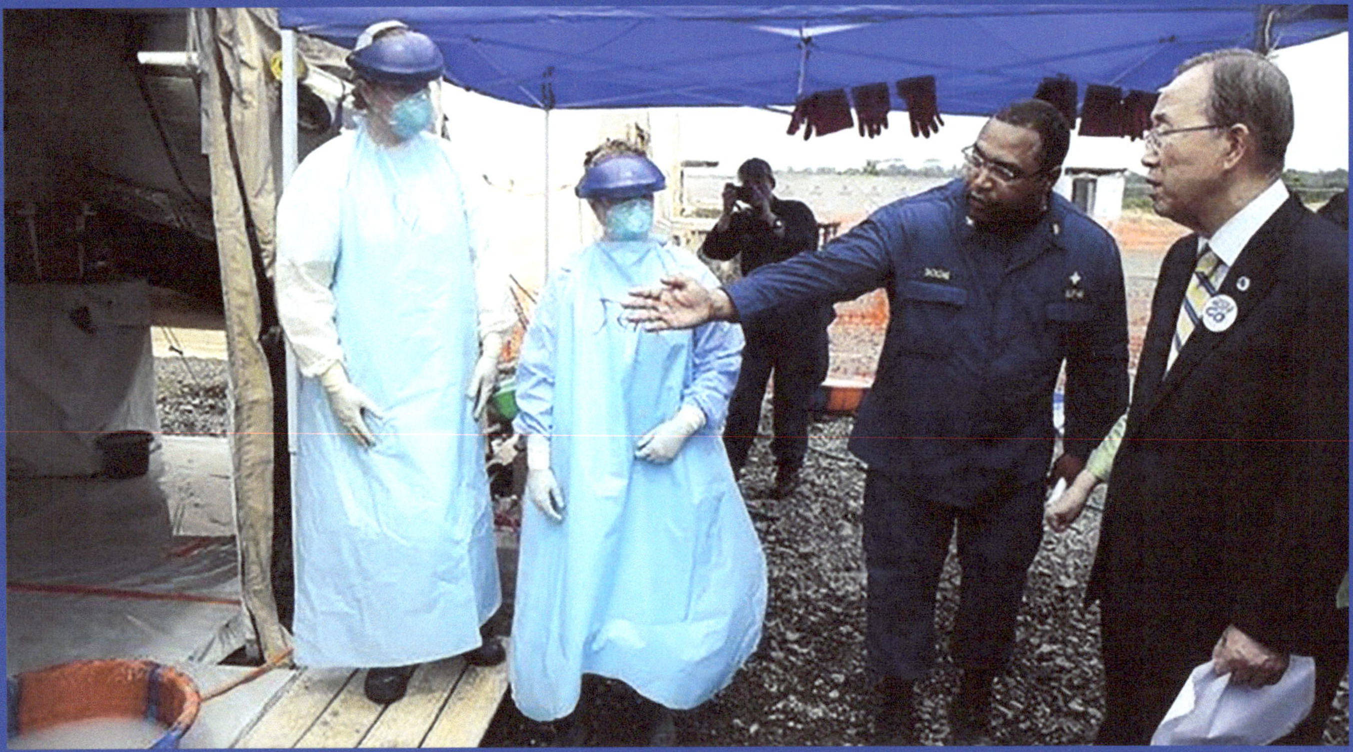

This photo was taken by United Nations (UN) photographer Evan Schneider and was shared across several international news media networks. CAPT Dickens, the Officer-in-Charge of the Monrovia Medical Unit (MMU) Team 2 *(pointing)*; LCDR Loveless; LCDR Bornermann; and LCDR Erb-Alvarez *(background)* provide a tour to UN Secretary-General Ban Ki-moon.

CONTENTS

SERVICE BEFORE SELF I

Foreword ix
Who We Are 10
An Introduction to Our Stories 13
The Mission 14

PREVENT 20

HSPAC Chair: Perspective as the Response Escalates 21
Stacey Atkins, PhD 22
CAPT Craig Wilkins 23
CAPT Amanda Dunnick 24
CDR Idongesit Essiet-Gibson 26
CDR Ibrahim Kamara 27
CDR Leslie Hausman 28
CDR Carolina Luna-Pinto 29
CDR Erica Sison 30
LCDR Sylvera Demas 31
LCDR Arthur Hurst 32
LT Allen Applegate 32
LT Jennifer Johnson 33
LT Samantha Morgan 34
LT Janesia Robbs 35

DETECT 36

HSPAC CHAIR: Perspective as the Response Begins 38
Todd Alspach, MOS, CLC (AMT), MT (ASCP) 39
Force Leadership Highlight LCDR Elizabeth DeGrange 40
CAPT Rendi Murphree 43
CAPT Angela K. Shen 44
CDR Christye Brown 46
CDR Jacinta Smith 47
CDR Christopher Duncan 49
CDR Thomas Christl 50
CDR Debra King 51
CDR Ericka Murray 52
LCDR Jennifer Cockrill 53
LCDR Elizabeth Garza 54
LCDR David Hunter 55

CONTENTS

LCDR Meredith Pyle ... 56
LCDR Osamede Onaghise ... 57
LT Roberto Garza ... 59
LT Khadar Diria ... 60
LT William Brown ... 61
LT Taran Pierce ... 63

RESPOND ... 65

HSPAC CHAIR: Perspective as the Mission Completes ... 66
Bobby Rasulnia, PhD, MPA, MPH, CHES ... 67
Force Leadership Highlight RADM Epi Elizondo ... 68
CAPT David de la Cruz ... 70
CAPT Robin MacGowan & LT Heather Joseph ... 72
CAPT Cynthia Spells ... 73
CAPT Robin Hunter Buskey ... 74
CAPT (Ret.) Dorothy Stephens ... 76
CAPT Robert Windom ... 77
CAPT Michael Schmoyer ... 78
CDR Kenneth Monahan ... 79
CDR Joseph Roth Jr. ... 80
CDR Charlene Majersky ... 81
CDR Torris Smith ... 82
CDR Tobey Manns Royal ... 83
CDRs Julie Chodacki and M. Sonsy Fermin ... 84
CDR Andrew Chen ... 85
CDR Erich Kleinschmidt ... 87
CDR Anthony Garza ... 88
CDR Jamie Seligman ... 89
CDR David Lau ... 91
CDR Tracy Pace ... 93
LCDR Jennifer Bornermann ... 94
LCDR Kate Migliaccio ... 95
LCDR Chris Poulson ... 96
LCDR Skip Payne ... 97
LCDR Matthew Johns ... 98
LCDR Philip Lafleur ... 99
LCDR Karen Forbes ... 100
LCDR Rafael Torres-Cruz ... 101
LCDR Julie Erb-Alvarez ... 102
LCDR Evelyn Seel ... 104

CONTENTS

LT Tracy Tilghman 104
LCDR Lorraine Williams 106
LT Jennifer Freiman 107
LT Anca Tabakova 108
LT Cody Thornton 109

MISSION COMPLETE 117

Presidential Unit Citation 119
Presidential Unit Citation Excerpt 125

HISTORY OF THE HEALTH SERVICES CATEGORY 129

HSPAC SEAL (2006–2019) 130

ACKNOWLEDGMENTS 131

INDEX AND LIST 132

Officer Index 133
Acronym List 134

Special Thanks to the HSO Special Edition Team!

Communications Advisor

CDR Elizabeth Garza, MPH, CPH

Readiness Advisor

CAPT Julie Erb-Alvarez, MPH, CPH

Project Team Lead & Co-Lead

LCDR Kimberly Goodwin, MPH
CDR Jessica Damon, MPH, MLS (ASCP)CM

Section Leads

Detect Section—*CDR Jessica Damon, MPH, MLS (ASCP)CM*
Prevent Section—*LCDR Lundy Patrick, MPH, MT (ASCP)*
Respond Section—*CDR Karen Forbes, MPA-S, PA-C*

Senior Editor

CAPT Kimberly McIntosh-Little, MBA, LNHA

Consulting Editor

CDR Kate Migliaccio Grabill, MPH

Visual Design Specialist

LCDR Mouhamed Halwani, MPH, MS, MB (ASCP) CM

This special edition would not have been possible without the guidance and leadership of:

Health Services Category, Chief Professional Officer

CAPT Jeanine Willis Marsh, DPM

2018 Chair, HSPAC

CAPT Carlos Bell, MPH, PMP, FAC-COR III

The HSO special edition Ebola team would like to extend heartfelt thanks to the officers who submitted personal stories and photographs from their deployment.

"Multidisciplinary in Approach, Connected by Service, Advancing Public Health."

FOREWORD

Everyone deserves to know about the USPHS Commissioned Corps of the US Public Health Service. So much of our country's public health—from just before the turn of the 20th century until the present day—has been impacted by this relatively small but mighty force of uniformed service officers.

In 2014, during the worst Ebola outbreak in documented history, the USPHS Commissioned Corps was called upon to respond. In arguably the most visible of multiple missions, the White House and National Security Council tasked the Corps to deploy to Liberia and create the Monrovia Medical Unit (MMU), staffing it with providers until Ebola was stopped at its source. It was a rare opportunity to help prevent a potential global pandemic and truly showcase our varied expertise and adaptability in an austere environment outside our nation's borders. It was also one of the first times in history where we as a uniformed service were able to function more independently as equal partners at the table with other essential stakeholders. In addition to the MMU, the Corps was involved in other Ebola-related missions that spanned both domestic and international responsibilities. Multiple missions required complex planning and coordination led by the State Department and the three host countries of Liberia, Sierra Leone, and Guinea. Partners included the Department of Defense, the World Health Organization, non-governmental organizations, and our colleagues in the Department of Health and Human Services and the Centers for Disease Control and Prevention.

The USPHS Commissioned Corps' Ebola response and the specific skill sets inherent to our Health Services Officers (HSOs) across all missions illuminated the bridges they can build with expertise in so many areas. Their ability to be nimble and flexible in response, to demonstrate resilience, to be culturally fluent, and to exemplify sheer determination amidst limited resources and training was admirable.

This collection of personal accounts represents a critical part of a larger team effort. These accounts should be treasured. I literally trusted many of them with our lives and personally relied on so many of them to fill essential roles. Because of their individual and collective courage and resilience, hundreds of new providers and responders followed into key areas of Liberia, which helped turn the tide of the Ebola response in West Africa. To each of the HSOs that successfully deployed, and to all the other officers that contributed directly (and indirectly) to the response, . . . bravo zulu! You will go down in our Corps' history with pride and distinction.

RADM Scott Giberson
Assistant U.S. Surgeon General
Commander, USPHS Commissioned Corps Ebola Response

WHO WE ARE

2010–2016 Health Services Category Chief Professional Officer

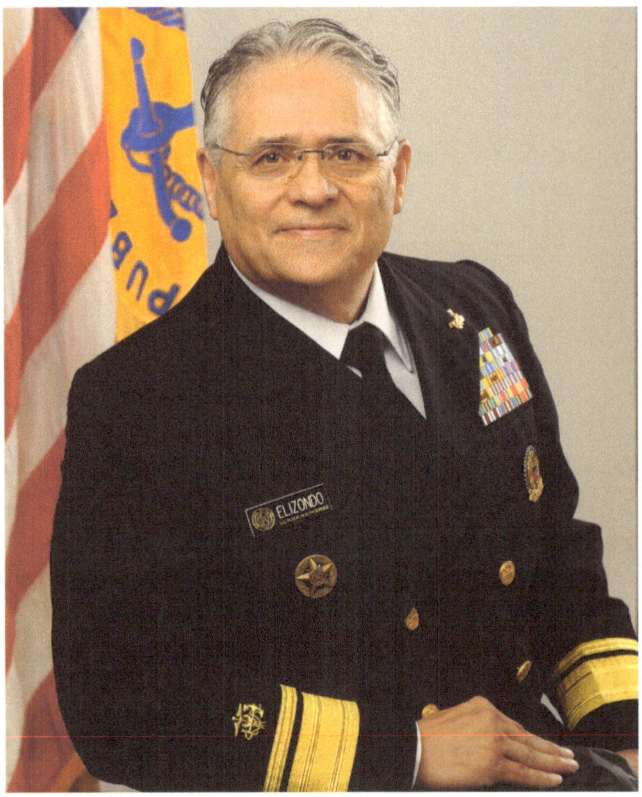

RADM (Ret.) Elizondo, PhD, PA-C, DFAAPA; HS CPO 2010–2016

Since its origin in 1798, men and women of the United States Public Health Service (USPHS) have served on the front lines of our nation's public health, protecting against the spread of disease. The Act for the Relief of Sick and Disabled Seamen, signed into law that year by President John Quincy Adams, established a series of marine hospitals to treat ill sailors returning from foreign ports and was extended the following year to likewise treat all US naval officials. In 1870, the administration of these hospitals was centralized via the creation of the Marine Hospital Service under the direction of a supervising surgeon (predecessor to the title of Surgeon General), the first of which was Dr. John Maynard Woodsworth. Dr. Woodsworth utilized military structure to organize and manage the physicians serving these hospitals. Industrialization continued to be a catalyst for the spread of disease, and in 1878 the US Congress established the National Quarantine Act, empowering the Marine Health Service with the charge to control the spread of disease outbreaks, greatly expanding its role. Finally, in 1889, Congress established the Commissioned Corps of the Marine Health Service organizing this deployable force of physicians under military ranks and pay equivalent to other United States uniformed services. The name was officially changed to Public Health Service (PHS) to match the expanded mission in 1912.

Today, the USPHS Commissioned Corps is one of eight uniformed services protecting the nation, along with the Army, Navy, Air Force, Marine Corps, Coast Guard, Space Force, and National Oceanic and Atmospheric Administration Commissioned Corps. The USPHS Commissioned Corps is the only uniformed service in the world dedicated to public health, authorized by Congress, commissioned by the president, and deployed by the secretary of the US Department of Health and Human Services (HHS). It is a unique, adaptable, mobile, and deployable force that stands ready to meet the public health needs of our nation and the world. The Commissioned Corps is part of the HHS, with 6,100 full time, highly qualified public health professionals. Officers serve underserved and vulnerable populations and engage in assignments that are isolated or hard to fill; hazardous; require availability twenty-four hours a day, seven days a week; and involve engagement with local communities and other uniformed services. In 2015, Commissioned Corps officers were assigned to nine US departments and over twenty federal government agencies, resulting in a broad and diverse public health network reaching across government to more than eight hundred duty stations worldwide. The responsibilities of the USPHS Commissioned Corps have grown through time to include the delivery of direct patient care to vulnerable communities impacted by poverty and rapid response to weather-related emergencies, terrorist attacks, and public health emergencies. USPHS Commissioned Corps officers often serve on the front lines in public health emergencies and crisis situations both foreign and domestic.

In recent times, the USPHS Commissioned Corps has deployed officers in response to significant events nationally and internationally, including deployments to West Africa in response to the 2014–2016 Ebola crisis. Over the last three decades, the Corps has deployed to terrorism responses including 9/11 and the Anthrax attacks of 2001; natural disasters such as hurricanes Sandy, Katrina, Wilma, Rita, Gustav, Ike, Harvey, Irma, and Maria and the Red River Flooding; humanitarian assistance missions including the Haiti earthquake, the Japan earthquake, Indonesian tsunamis, Operation Lone Star in south Texas, and the Unaccompanied Children Mission; reconstruction and stabilization in Iraq and Afghanistan; and public health crises responses to situations including H1N1, Saipan health system, suicide clusters in Indian Health Service (IHS), Zika virus, Ebola virus, the opioid epidemic, and the COVID-19 pandemic.

The Commissioned Corps was particularly affected by the international deployment of officers in response to the 2014–2016 Ebola crisis. This was the first deployment where the Commissioned Corps operated as an independent uniformed asset (in contrast to being subsumed by the operational response of the Department of Defense) and was the only US government asset to provide direct patient care to healthcare providers with Ebola in West Africa. The Monrovia Medical Unit (MMU) provided clinical care to local health professionals infected with the Ebola virus. The first team of officers arrived on October 27, 2014, and accepted their first patient on November 12. The facility completed its mission and was decommissioned on May 1, 2015.

This book highlights the third-largest category in the USPHS Commissioned Corps: Health Services. Many health services officers (HSOs) served in a variety of capacities during the Ebola response. Some officers served as part of the response leadership within the US Embassy in Monrovia, Liberia and collaborated directly with the US Agency for International Development Disaster Assistance Response Team (DART) and the Ministry of Health (MOH) of Liberia. Others deployed to airports to assist with enhanced Ebola Virus Disease (EVD) screening operations for passengers arriving from the three Ebola-affected countries. The majority of officers worked in the MMU as administrators, laboratory technologists, physician assistants, and mental health providers, and all played a role in training Liberian health professionals to operate the MMU and its equipment upon their departure for use in any future outbreaks. The medical symposium at the Monrovia Medical School held by MMU Team 4 was important to both the Commissioned Corps and the MOH of Liberia. It was attended by MOH leadership, providers, medical students, survivors, deployed officers, and the US Surgeon General Vice Admiral Murthy Vivek, MD, MBA.

Health Services is one of eleven professional categories of the USPHS. HSOs contribute vitally to the health of the nation and are an invaluable resource to the Office of the Surgeon General, USPHS, other governmental agencies, and the American public. As of 2020, there are close to 1,200 HSOs from a wide variety of disciplines. They hold qualifying degrees from accredited clinical, scientific, technical, and administrative programs. HSOs represent over fifty disciplines, including biological, physical and environmental sciences, optometry, clinical psychology, social work, podiatry, medical technology, dental hygiene, medical records administration, physician assistance, information technology, global health, health education, healthcare administration, and other public health specialties. The HSO motto—Multidisciplinary in Approach, Connected by Service, Advancing Public Health—attests to the wide range of skills and experience possessed by this multidisciplinary team of officers and to their pride and commitment to serving in the Commissioned Corps.

As a former chief professional officer (CPO) of health services officers, it was an honor to serve as one of four commanders of this historic event. It was equally satisfying to work directly with the US ambassador, DART, the MOH of Liberia, and representatives from both the US Army and the Centers for Disease Control and Prevention (CDC). Most important, however, was witnessing officers caring for fellow human beings across the Atlantic Ocean with utmost compassion and professionalism. Equally gratifying was the profound appreciation of the Liberian people and their healthcare team members.

Much was learned! Much was achieved! Much more was left to do! Onward and upward!

Rear Admiral (ret.) Epifanio (Epi) Elizondo
Retired U.S. Assistant Surgeon General, USPHS
Former Regional Health Administrator for Region VI
(TX, NM, OK, AR, and LA)

AN INTRODUCTION TO OUR STORIES

2018 Health Services Professional Advisory Committee (HSPAC) Chair

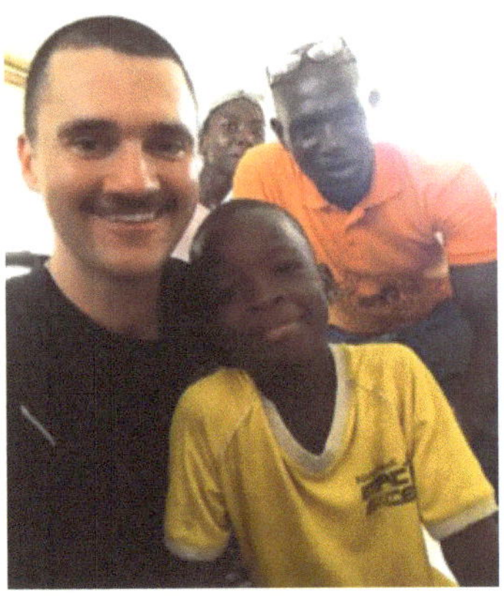

In February 2015, Monrovia Medical Unit (MMU) Team 2 returned home to the US, having successfully completed our mission of providing care, compassion, and comfort to the people of Liberia. All of us have experienced a range of emotions after homecomings from deployments, but this one was different. I suspect many of us feel the same way, even after four years. I can still remember the humbling feeling of having served as Team 2's public information officer (PIO) and the incredible sense of belonging and purpose that accompanied our critical work. It was the privilege of a lifetime to serve alongside so many talented and dedicated fellow USPHS Commissioned Corps officers.

While it could be argued that even the most experienced responders among us were not completely prepared for this specific deployment and the conditions on the ground, I am particularly proud of all of the junior officers and those officers who deployed for the first time. In every situation, these individuals exceeded expectations and represented the Commissioned Corps with grace, professionalism, determination, compassion, and courage.

As I write this introductory passage, I am reminded of many powerful encounters and emotions. One in particular will always stay with me: A few weeks after we arrived, and the daily routine of our work was setting in, I remember making a visit to a local orphanage that had taken in children whose parents, family, and friends had passed away from Ebola. It was Christmas Eve. Given the devastation these children had experienced, I was unsure what to expect. To my surprise, the children greeted us with beaming smiles and joyous laughter—grateful and excited to welcome their new visitors. In an instant, my entire mood changed, and I saw the hope and love that our officers provided to these children. I saw the best of the USPHS that afternoon at that orphanage, and in every day before and after.

Over six hundred officers deployed to serve the people of Liberia during the 2014 Ebola outbreak response, and many of them were fellow health services officers. On behalf of those officers, and with a great sense of comradery and pride, I am honored to introduce this health services officer (HSO)–focused deployment book.

I want to personally thank every officer who deployed in theater to West Africa and every officer who worked to support the deployment stateside, including officers who stepped up to ensure the continuity of our work across agencies. This book is a reflection of all of you, and I am grateful to all HSOs who took the time to submit their stories, photos, quotes, and memories. Lastly, this book would not be possible without the incredible members of the HSO Special Edition Team who have spent countless hours putting this important piece of history together for the Commissioned Corps. Thank you to everyone.

Forever grateful,

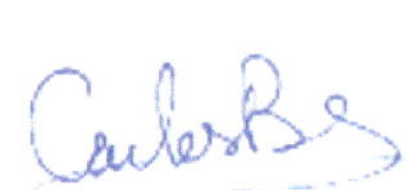

CAPT Carlos Bell
MMU Team 2, PIO/LNO
2018 Chair, HSPAC

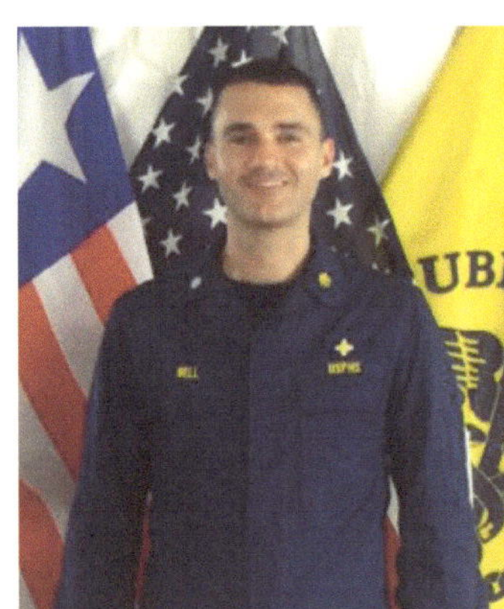

THE MISSION

The 2014–2016 Ebola Virus Disease (EVD) epidemic in West Africa required a massive international response to assist the affected countries. It tested the world's readiness to respond to global health emergencies. In 2014, the USPHS Commissioned Corps was called by President Obama to respond to the Ebola epidemic in West Africa. Assistant Secretary for Health and Human Services Sylvia Burwell, BA, authorized activation and deployment of the Corps in support of the department's role in the US government response to the Ebola outbreak in West Africa. The first case was reported in Guinea in March 2014, and the disease spread quickly in the neighboring countries of Liberia and Sierra Leone. Over the span of a year, the Ebola epidemic caused more than ten times as many cases of Ebola as the combined total of previously-reported Ebola outbreaks. As the outbreak became more widespread, travel-associated cases appeared in Nigeria, Mali, Senegal, and even countries outside of Africa, including the US. Overall, nine countries reported cases of Ebola; more than 28,616 people had suspected, probable, or confirmed Ebola; and 11,310 died1, these numbers were likely even higher, as many cases went undiagnosed and unreported.

> **"Fighting this disease had to be more than a national security priority but an example of American leadership. After all, whenever and wherever a disaster of disease strikes, the world looks to us to lead, and because of extraordinary people, we have risen to the challenge. All of you represent what is best about America and what is possible when we lead."**
>
> —*President Barack Obama*
> (February 2015)

The Ebola epidemic was one of the most challenging global public health emergencies in recent times. Not only was this epidemic unprecedented; so was the public health response. Together, our Commissioned Corps officers and officials, the Centers for Disease Control and Prevention (CDC), military personnel, and teams from other federal agencies were a part of the largest-ever US government response to a global health crisis.

As a result, for the first time in our history, the Commissioned Corps received a Presidential Unit Citation (PUC). The president of the United States, who is also the Commissioned Corps' commander-in-chief, presented the PUC to the Commissioned Corps for its response to the Ebola outbreak in West Africa after the successful return of the four Monrovia Medical Unit (MMU) teams from Liberia. As written in the citation, "Commissioned Corps officers were the only United States government asset to provide direct patient care to healthcare workers with Ebola in West Africa." President Obama presented the PUC during an Oval Office ceremony on September 24, 2015. The event was even more distinctive, as Oval Office ceremonies for unit awards rarely occur. The citation was awarded to all Corps officers for "extraordinary courage and the highest level of performance in action throughout the response to the Ebola outbreak." Whether deployed to West Africa, staffing quarantine stations or emergency operations centers domestically, or back-filling positions, this was an all-Corps response.

RADM Scott Giberson, Acting Deputy Surgeon General, led the mission in Liberia to care for healthcare workers at the MMU so they in turn could care for Ebola patients throughout the region. Over two hundred officers voluntarily deployed to the MMU in Liberia. Over the course of the seven months, four teams of officers were created, consisting of seventy to eighty officers

1— https://apps.who.int/iris/bitstream/handle/10665/208883/ebolasitrep_10Jun2016_eng.pdf;sequence=1

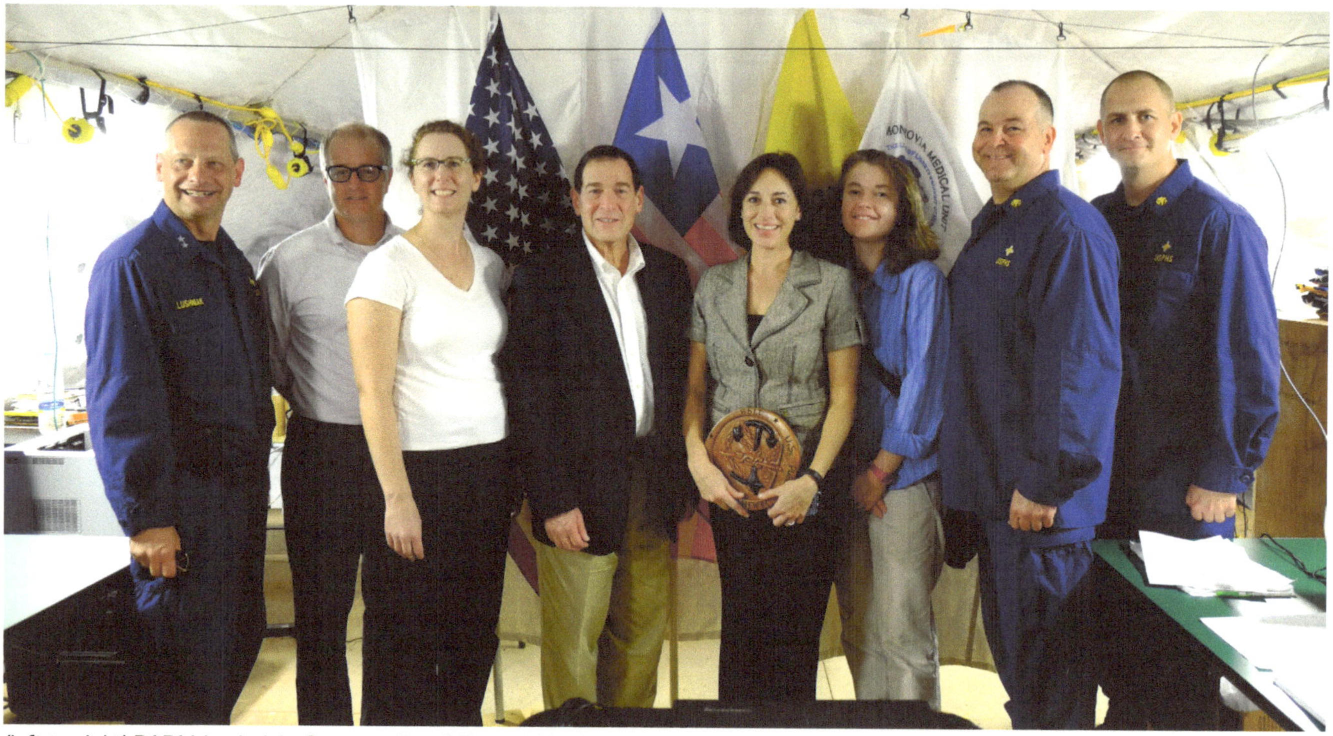

(left to right) RADM Lushniak, Commanding Officer (CO) USPHS Liberia (Jan-Feb 2015); Mr. Doug Mercado, United States Agency for International Development (USAID) Disaster Assistance Response Team (DART); Carol Han, US Embassy Public Affairs; Ambassador Kolker, Assistant Secretary Global Affairs; Dr. Desalvo, Assistant Secretary for Health; Ms. Dawn O'Connell, Deputy Chief of Staff for the Health and Human Services (HHS); CAPT Coppola, MMU Officer-in-Charge (OIC); CAPT Boyd, MMU Deputy Officer-in-Charge (DOIC). Photo taken in MMU Command Tent.

on each team. The USPHS Commissioned Corps staffed the MMU—a twenty-five-bed, state-of-the-art hospital—the only unit of its kind in the region that provided care to healthcare workers who may have been infected with the Ebola virus.

"This part of the mission is critically important, because healthcare workers are at higher risk of infection. It is really important that we provide them with quality care, first and foremost because they offer hope and healing to patients throughout the region, and secondly because we want to make sure that healthcare workers throughout the world know there is a resource for them if they get sick so that they will continue to lend their hand."

Dr. Karen DeSalvo
Acting Assistant Secretary for Health

"We are in West Africa to offer help, healing, and hope—continuing the legacy of our Corps and our country. When our neighbors need us most, we Americans open our hearts and extend our hands—regardless of whether they live in places near or far. In this sense we are there to be hope multipliers. . . . To save lives, we need safe facilities and safe equipment, and most importantly, we need to keep the people safe who are doing the saving."

LCDR Kate Migliaccio
Senior Public Information Officer (PIO), Office of the Assistant Secretary for Health

Outside of the MMU mission, the Corps had officers supporting a wide range of other Ebola-related mission assignments. Officers deployed, not only through the Commissioned Corps Headquarters' Readiness and Deployment Branch (formerly known as RedDOG), but also with the CDC, the National Institutes of Health (NIH), and the Office of the Assistant Secretary for Preparedness and Response (ASPR) both stateside and in Africa. As the Ebola epidemic involved a viral disease pathogen, the CDC formed the lead federal agency in the US government response to this threat. At the peak of the response, the CDC maintained approximately two hundred staff per day in West Africa and approximately four hundred staff per day at its Atlanta headquarters dedicated to the response. Overall, approximately 1,897 CDC staff were deployed to international and US locations, for approximately 110,000 total work days, and more than four thousand CDC staff worked as part of the response. In addition to their work in West Africa, CDC staff played a critical role protecting the United States by aiding state and local health departments in their preparedness activities and their response to the country's first imported Ebola cases. The CDC helped international, federal, and state partners establish airport risk assessment of travelers departing and arriving from affected countries, monitored travelers and other potentially exposed persons for twenty-one days2, and helped hospitals across the country prepare to manage a possible case of Ebola through intensive training and preparedness activities. A large number of the CDC staff involved in the response were Commissioned Corps officers. Through the CDC's collaboration with national and international partners steady improvement was made in the areas of disease surveillance, contact tracing, diagnostic testing, community engagement and ownership, infection prevention and control, border health, emergency management, and vaccine evaluation. The 2014–2016 Ebola epidemic was the largest emergency response in CDC history.

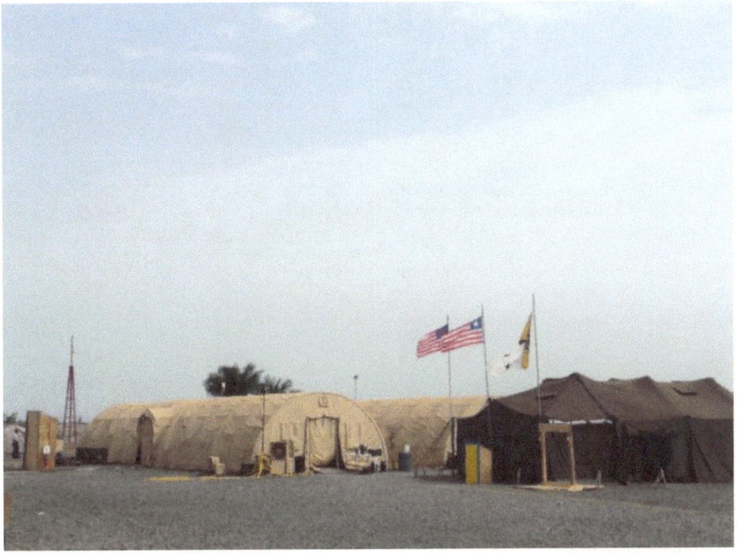

Other notable federal entities involved in the response included the ASPR/Biomedical Advanced Research and Development Authority (BARDA), the Food and Drug Administration (FDA), and the NIH. BARDA received $157 million through a FY 2015 Omnibus Appropriations Bill3 that included resources to manufacture vaccines and synthetic therapeutics for use in clinical trials against Ebola virus. The NIH received $238 million in funding advanced clinical trials to evaluate the safety and efficacy of investigational vaccines and therapeutics. The FDA received $25 million which included funding for development, review, regulation, and post-market surveillance of an Ebola vaccine and therapeutics. The FDA worked with product sponsors, US government funding agencies, and international partners to clarify data, clinical studies, and regulatory requirements necessary to facilitate the development and availability of the most promising vaccines and therapeutics that could potentially mitigate the Ebola virus outbreak. The FDA used its flexible regulatory framework, such as issuing emergency use authorizations, to make available investigational in vitro diagnostics needed to detect Ebola in West Africa.

According to the CDC, a total of 28,616 cases of EVD were identified during the 2014–2016 Ebola epidemic in West African countries of Sierra Leone, Guinea, and Liberia. Of these identified cases, 11,310 deaths were reported. Due to the high rate of contractibility during the care and handling of patients, healthcare workers in these countries were disproportionately affected. Liberia reported a loss of nearly 8 percent of its clinical care

2—https://www.cdc.gov/vhf/ebola/exposure/monitoring-and-movement-of-persons-with-exposure.html

3—U.S. Congress. Public Law No: 113-235; December 16, 2014.

providers at a time when the demands for care were extraordinarily high. Caring for these healthcare providers and preventing further loss of life and impairment to the overall healthcare system was the unique mission of the USPHS Commissioned Corps. Additionally, during the course of this crisis, eleven patients received treatment in the United States, with four of these patients developing signs of illness after arriving on US soil. However, all instances of exposure were isolated to the West African continent. In part this was also due to the intensity of the response and the dedication of the officers serving on the frontlines and at the ports of entry here at home.

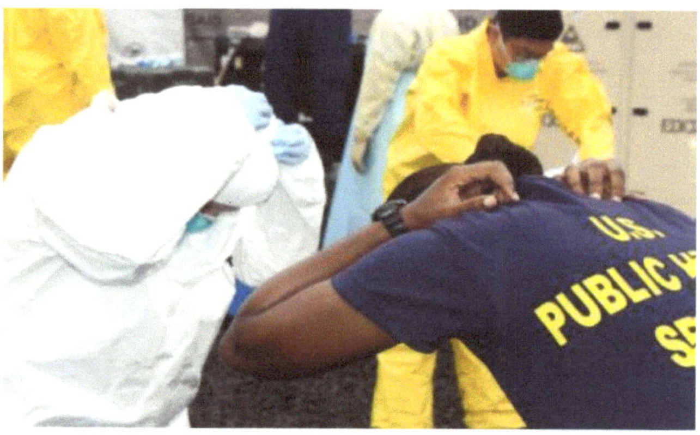

MMU Team 4 is instructed on proper safety of doffing an officer who has come out of the hot-zone. Proper process of decontamination and step-by-step action for removal of personal protective equipment (PPE) is critical in the doffing area to prevent accidental contamination.

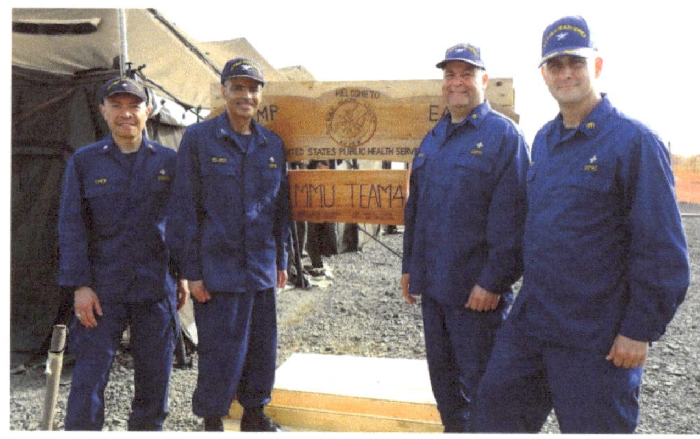

(left to right) CDR Chen, Deputy Officer-in-Charge (DOIC); CAPT Belardo, Officer-in-Charge (OIC); CAPT Coppola, OIC; and CAPT Boyd, DOIC, posing by the Camp Eason sign prior to the change of command from MMU Team 3 to MMU Team 4.

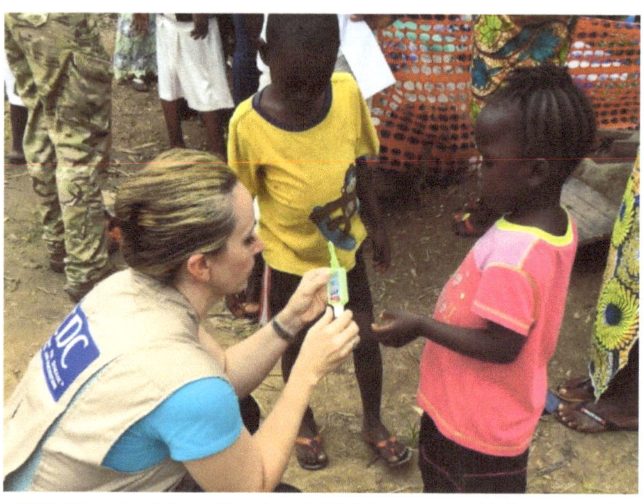

LCDR Weagle visits with a local child during a multisite quarantine release ceremony in Mamusa village, Marampa Chiefdom, of Port Loko, Sierra Leone, on August 5, 2015. LCDR Weagle deployed in support of the CDC Ebola response in West Africa, where she was selected as one of only four District Field Coordinators. As CDC Port Loko District field coordinator, she was responsible for surveillance, epidemiological and humanitarian efforts allocated to support over five hundred thousand residents.

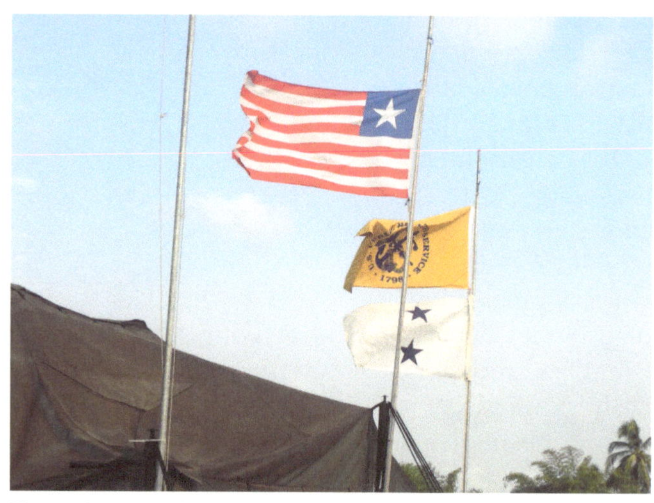

Flags raised over Camp Eason

"Seeing CAPT Cal Edwards (MMU Commanding Officer) come down the steps from the large chartered jet leading the Commissioned Corps Ebola Response Team truly ignited my emotions. CAPT Edwards rendered his salute and essentially reported his team for duty to me. With CAPT Reed, CAPT Schmoyer, and CDRs Davis and Gnipp standing with me, LCDR Kate Migliaccio snapped this picture. We went directly from the airport for a very short drive to the MMU. At that time, all seventy officers were inside the MMU with the generators humming, as well as a mix of some United States Agency for International Development (USAID) personnel, Department of Defense (DOD) personnel, and media journalists. It was time for a brief speech to welcome the team and set the tone. I have given many talks and speeches across my career, but for the next twelve minutes, no words meant more to me than what I attempted to convey to the team that their specific mission, their specific and critical piece of this global response, will turn the tide of this outbreak. Ebola has taken a piece of Liberia from its people. We, the United States Public Health Service (USPHS) Commissioned Corps, were called upon by our leadership to take that back."

Acting Deputy Surgeon General RADM Scott Giberson
(October 2014)

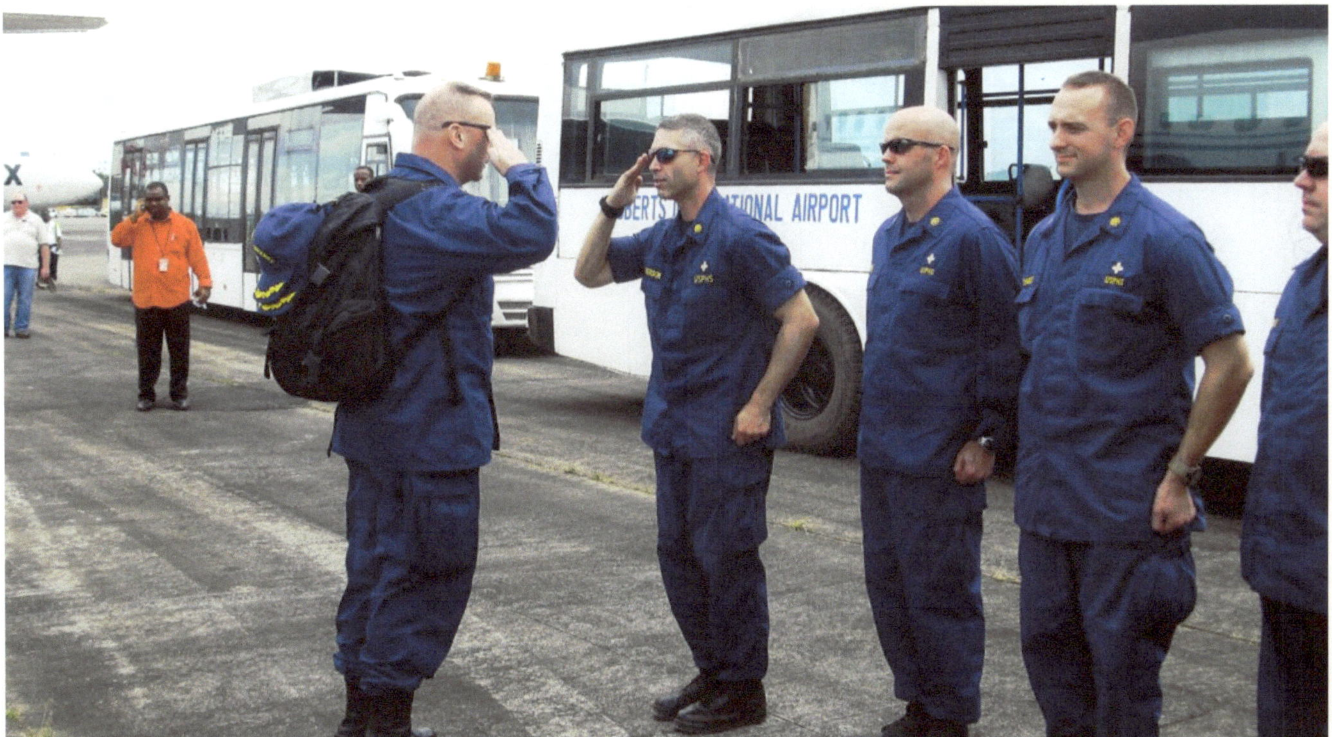

CAPT Edwards salutes RADM Giberson on the airport runway in front of the airport shuttle buses poised and ready to transport the team of officers.

Disease prevention is the first pillar in the Global Health Security framework and it encompasses the actions, innovations, and coordinated efforts specifically targeted toward keeping healthy people healthy. The objective of disease prevention is to reduce the incidence of disease in a given population. In the context of the Ebola outbreak, where the virus was already present in the initial population, activities supporting reduction in further spread included vaccine development and human vaccine trials, health education to promote safe community and medical practices, and health messaging to decrease fear and encourage resilience in affected populations. Officers supported these activities both stateside and abroad, working seamlessly with federal and international agencies, community health networks, and local responders to control spread of the Ebola virus through implementation of scientific and strategic based prevention strategies.

The following stories have been selected to demonstrate the breadth and depth of this work. The section is introduced by the 2015 HSPAC Chair, CAPT Stacey Atkins who led the HSPAC as the response activation rapidly escalated while simultaneously deploying out of country. In addition, it features a Force Leadership Highlight by CAPT Craig Wilkins who served as a liaison officer for the CDC coordinating epidemiology and surveillance activities with strategic partners. These two features are intended to set the stage for the stories that follow. The officer accounts of their work and the impact of participating in these prevention efforts are presented following military custom with the highest ranking officers given the floor first in presentation. Some stories included in the section may have activities that span all three pillars of Global Health Security (prevent, detect, respond) but they have been placed here for the dramatic representation of prevention strategies.

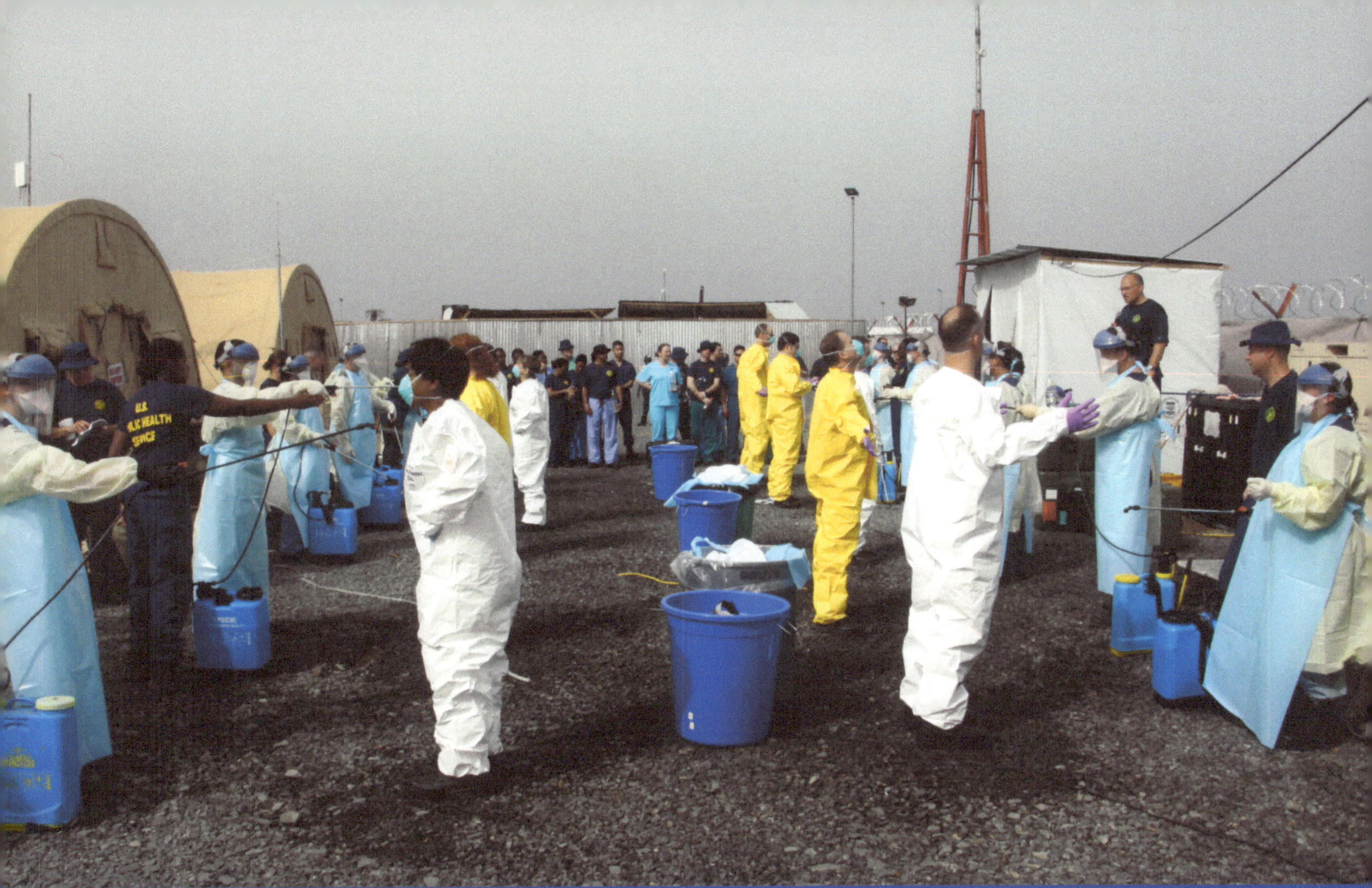

PREVENT

"A critical goal of this mission was to rapidly prevent further spread of the virus. To accomplish this goal, health services officers were assigned to both the austere environs of the African continent and domestically at key points of entry in the United States. In addition, many officers served within their respective agency assignments to support the containment activities of the mission. Whether they were serving on the front lines, providing prophylactic treatment in clinical settings, developing a new vaccine, providing education to the most vulnerable, or providing preventative care here at home to the officers prior to and following deployment, these officers were the "tip of the sword" in the fight against Ebola."

Lundy Patrick, MPH, MT (ASCP)
LCDR, USPHS

HSPAC Chair: Perspective as the Response Escalates

CAPT Stacey Atkins shares, "I imagine that I speak for many of us that serve in the elite cadre of officers in the USPHS Commissioned Corps when I say that, whether domestically or internationally, we served our country with great honor, pride, and distinction. This was the first time that we functioned as an independent uniformed asset of the United States government within the Health and Human Services (HHS), instead of being a subordinate entity of the Department of Defense (DOD)." The Commissioned Corps mission from the White House was to roster healthcare professionals, administrators, and clinical staff to manage and operate a twenty-five–bed Ebola Treatment Unit (ETU) in Monrovia, Liberia. The Monrovia Medical Unit (MMU) provided high-level Ebola treatment for national and international healthcare workers so they, in turn, could care for Ebola patients throughout the region, bolstering international confidence to respond, provide hope, and offer a commitment to care for those who were fighting Ebola on the front lines. Starting in October 2014, teams of seventy officers deployed to the Centers for Disease Control and Prevention (CDC) Ebola-related training in Anniston, Alabama. Officers received textbook, mock, and hands-on training to ensure sufficient knowledge of Ebola and its transmission routes to work safely and efficiently in a well-designed ETU. Four teams deployed in response to this mission.

> **"It was especially exciting to see how the officers in our category harkened the call to duty to assist the individuals in West Africa."**
>
> —*Stacey Atkins, PhD*
> *CAPT, USPHS*
> Health Services Professional Advisory Committee (HSPAC) Chair, 2015

CAPT Atkins recalls, "Although I was the HSPAC chair-elect at the onset of the call for volunteers, there was never any doubt in my mind that I would volunteer myself. I am of the mindset that you do not have the people you serve alongside do anything that you would not do yourself. Although I was not sure how I was going to deploy as part of the MMU Team 2 Command Staff as the administration and finance section chief and still uphold my responsibilities as the incoming Professional Advisory Committee (PAC) chair, once deployed, it all came together. Teamwork definitely makes the dream work! I would like to acknowledge all of the HSPAC subcommittee chairs, Past PAC chairs, and each officer for ensuring that we exercised '1.2.3. The Power of the PAC!' during this time." CAPT Atkins deployed with outstanding leaders who were not only passionate about advancing the public health of the nation but also about HSPAC. Many officers offered their support and assistance in and out of country. The first HSPAC meeting of 2015 was even hosted from Liberia with the help of technology and officers that were stateside. An unprecedented number of officers participated in that meeting. CAPT Atkins reflects, "It was also especially exciting to see how the officers in our category harkened to the call of duty to assist the individuals in West Africa. Non-deployed health services officers made a significant contribution to the response by staying behind to serve in-country in taking up deployed colleagues' workload. Many officers also served in Liberia in the MMU with a responsibility for delivering state-of-the-art care to healthcare workers potentially and actually infected with the Ebola virus. In addition to the MMU, some officers were deployed and served with the CDC and the National Institutes of Health (NIH). Our category leadership was on the front line of the epidemic as our former chief professional officer (CPO) RADM Epi Elizondo (Ret.) served on MMU Team 4, which was the team that transitioned responsibility to the Liberian government. I would like to acknowledge each of the health services officers (HSOs) that served our Corps and country with pride and distinction as Ebola fighters!"

Stacey Atkins, PhD

CAPT, USPHS
HSPAC Chair, 2015

Dr. Stacey Atkins, also referred to as CAPT Stacey (0-6) Atkins, received her commission into the USPHS Health Services category in 2000. She has served her country on a number of deployments, including 911/Ground Zero, New York City (2001); Hurricane Anthrax, Washington, DC (2001); Hurricane Isabel, Tidewater Area, Virginia (2003); Hurricane Katrina, New Orleans Louisiana (2005); Tropical Storm Irene, New York (2011); the Sandy Hook School Incident, Newtown, Connecticut, (2012); MMU Team 2, Monrovia, Liberia (2014); and the Flint, Mississippi, Water Crisis (2016). Prior to joining the USPHS, CAPT Atkins worked for state government family service organizations and various non-profit faith-based organizations. CAPT Atkins has served in serval leadership roles in various operating divisions within HHS and DOD and has received several awards in recognition of her contributions for promoting health and wellness. Presently, CAPT Atkins is assigned to HHS, Health Resources and Services Administration (HRSA), Bureau of Health Workforce, Division of Health Careers and Financial Support, where she serves as the deputy director. CAPT Atkins earned a bachelor of science from the University of the District of Columbia. She later earned a master of social work degree from Howard University. CAPT Atkins earned her doctorate of philosophy in human services and behavioral studies from Capella University.

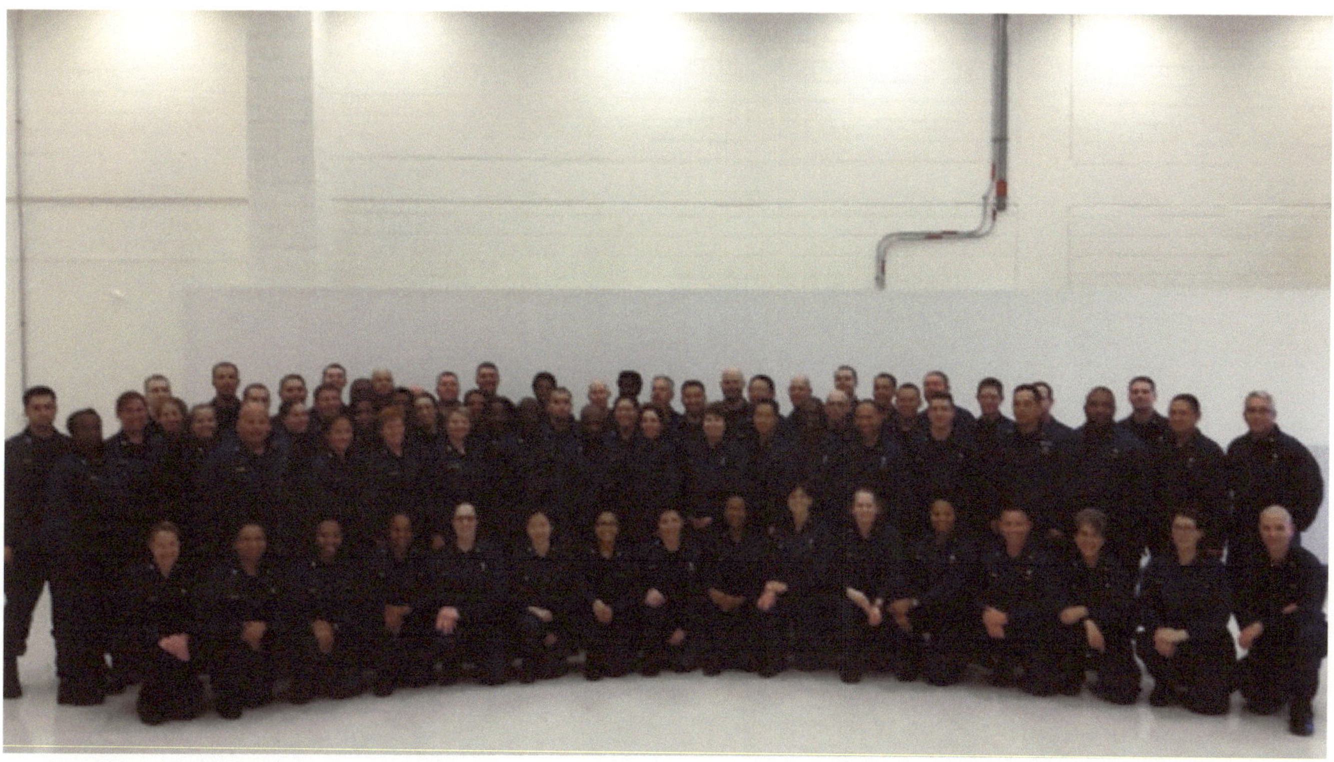

CAPT Atkins with MMU Team 2.

CAPT Craig Wilkins

"One of the most meaningful aspects of deployment was the opportunity to meet Ebola survivors and listen to their stories of survival and how some of them dealt with being ostracized within their own families and communities."

—Craig Wilkins, MPH

CAPT Craig Wilkins was deployed to Guinea from January to March 2015 in support of the Ebola response in West Africa. CAPT Wilkins was selected to serve as the Centers for Disease Control and Prevention (CDC) liaison officer to the Disaster Assistance Response Team (DART), the Office of US Foreign Disaster Assistance, and the United States Agency for International Development (USAID).

CAPT Wilkins' deployment responsibilities included leading CDC's collaborative efforts with DART on identifying Ebola partner issues and needs while providing key inputs for DART program planning for the response in Guinea. His priority issues for the response focused on infection prevention and control (IPC), epidemiology and surveillance, and communication and health promotion. He also conducted surveillance and a needs assessment for the establishment of Prefecture Emergency Operations Centers in regions of the country that had the highest cases of Ebola.

CAPT Wilkins reflects, "One of the most meaningful aspects of deployment was the opportunity to meet Ebola survivors and listen to their stories of survival and how some of them dealt with being ostracized within their own families and communities."

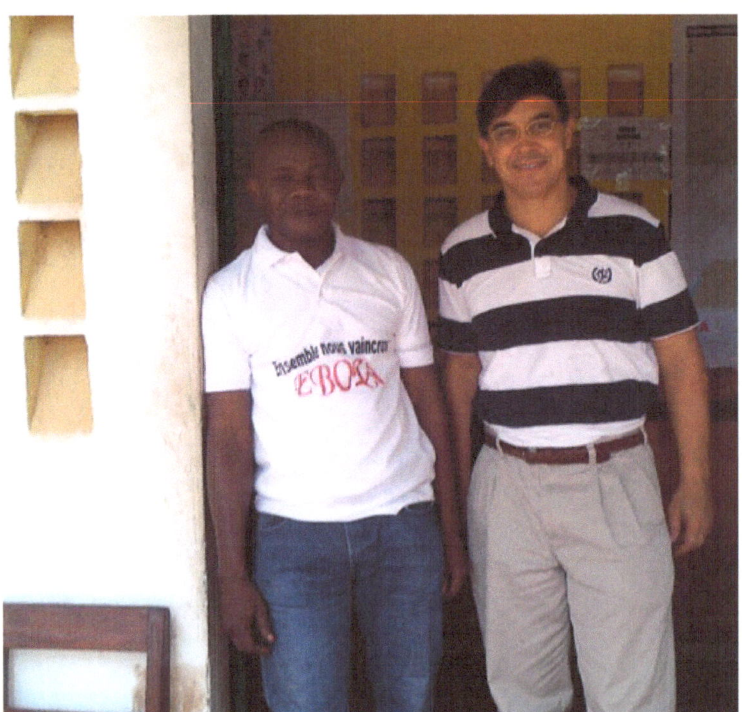

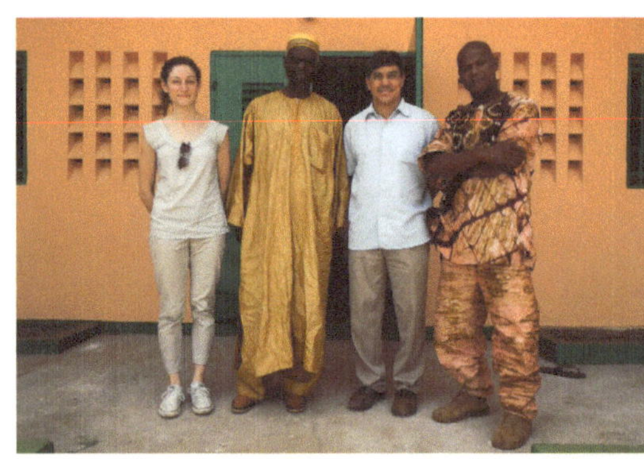

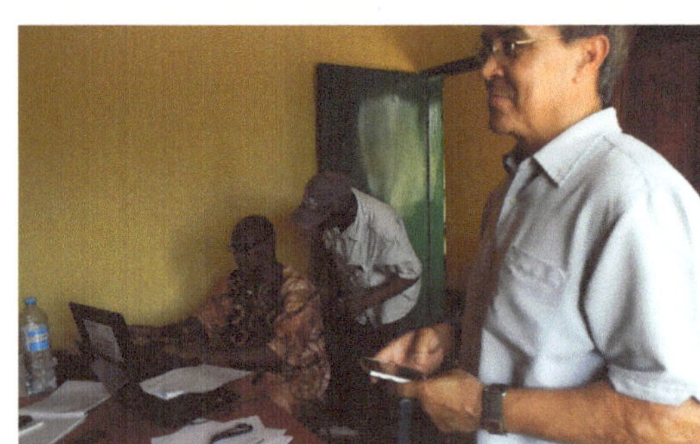

(far left) CAPT Wilkins is pictured *(right)* standing beside a local Ebola healthcare worker. *(top right)* CAPT Wilkins is featured here, third from the left, with Dubreka Health center staff. *(bottom left)* CAPT Wilkins participates in a meeting with the Dubreka Health Staff.

CAPT Amanda Dunnick

"This deployment was a highlight in my United States Public Health Service (USPHS) career, providing frontline public health to those in need. It taught me that we all have something to offer this world, and mine is to try and make it a little bit better each and every day."

—Amanda Dunnick, MPH

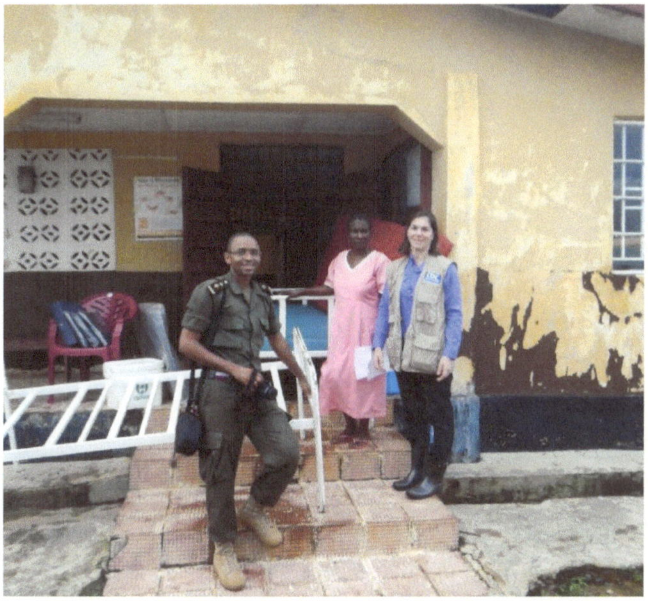

CAPT Dunnick *(right)* delivering supplies to public health units.

CAPT Amanda Dunnick's first trip to Africa occurred from September to October 2015. She deployed not to a large city but rather up-country in Sierra Leone, leading the Centers for Disease Control and Prevention (CDC) Port Loko infection prevention and control (IPC) activities. CAPT Dunnick discovered her up-country assignment on departure day. Of talking with her predecessor, CAPT Dunnick says, "She told me I needed a mini crockpot, canned soup, and more, or else I would starve. My first thought was 'What am I getting myself into?'" At the airport, CAPT Dunnick discovered a fellow CDC colleague was on the same flight—good news! He had been to Africa before, provided background to the situation, and relieved her fears. Next came recovery from jet lag, safety brief, and currency exchange; then off to Port Loko.

IPC has many aspects that involve changing lifestyle and practices. The CDC's main objective was to conduct regular assessments of the public health units (PHU) to ensure they were following proper IPC guidelines, such as handwashing upon entering the PHU, separate Ebola assessment area, disposal of waste, and more. Most days, CAPT Dunnick would travel to the PHUs throughout the district, conducting assessments and talking with the providers about what was working well and their needs. The PHUs had a good handle of the IPC procedures; however, they would frequently run out of soap and hand sanitizer, and most had wooden beds and fabric mattresses. It became clear that supplies could be key. CAPT Dunnick worked with the District Health Management Team to discover a cache of vinyl-covered foam mattresses and metal frames. In a few weeks, they delivered about fifty new beds throughout Port Loko. It was amazing to see how thrilled the local healthcare providers were to receive these basic supplies and know what a difference it would make.

CAPT Dunnick also worked with the vaccine trial team, which used local staff to administer pregnancy tests and vaccines. CAPT Dunnick would train the providers on how to implement IPC measures when handling urine samples, coming into contact with the patients, and disposing of used needles. The team so appreciated learning from the trainings that they were implemented at future vaccine trail dates.

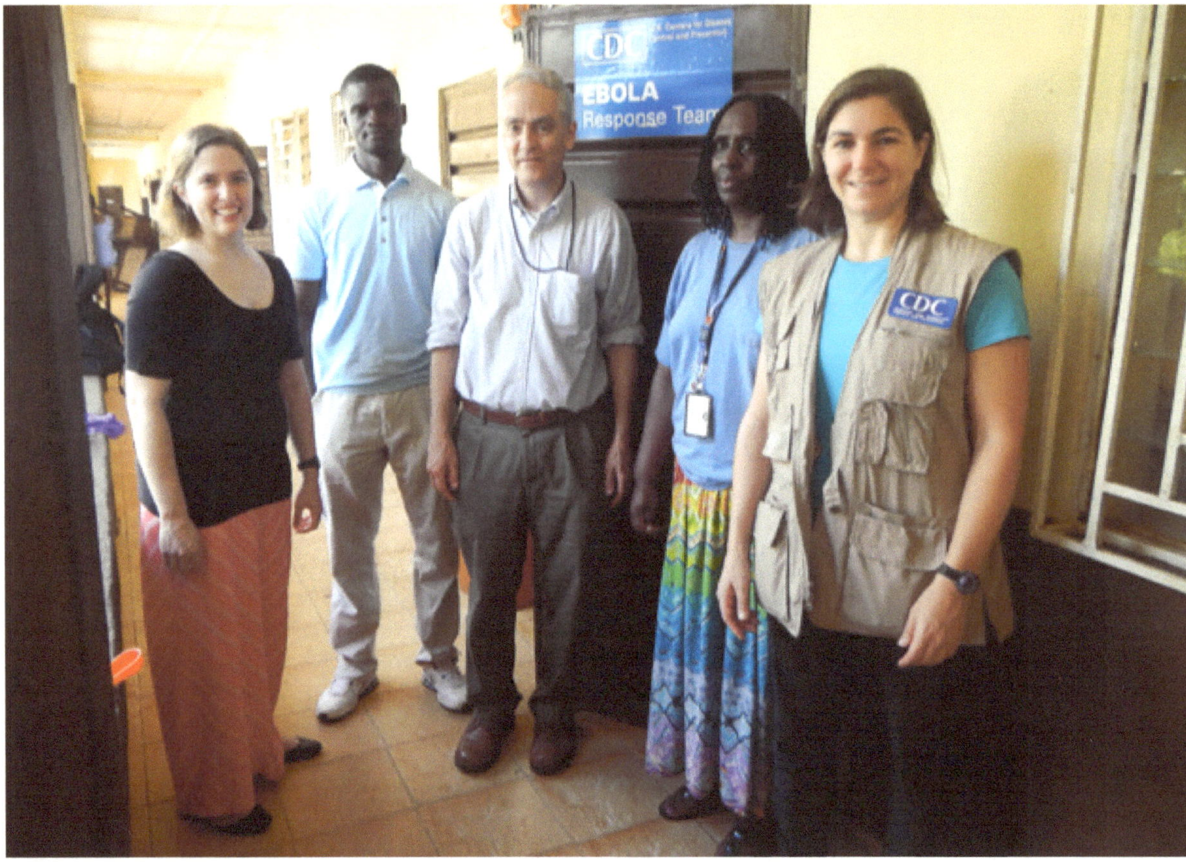

CAPT Dunnick *(right)* wearing CDC vest with the CDC Port Loko Team.

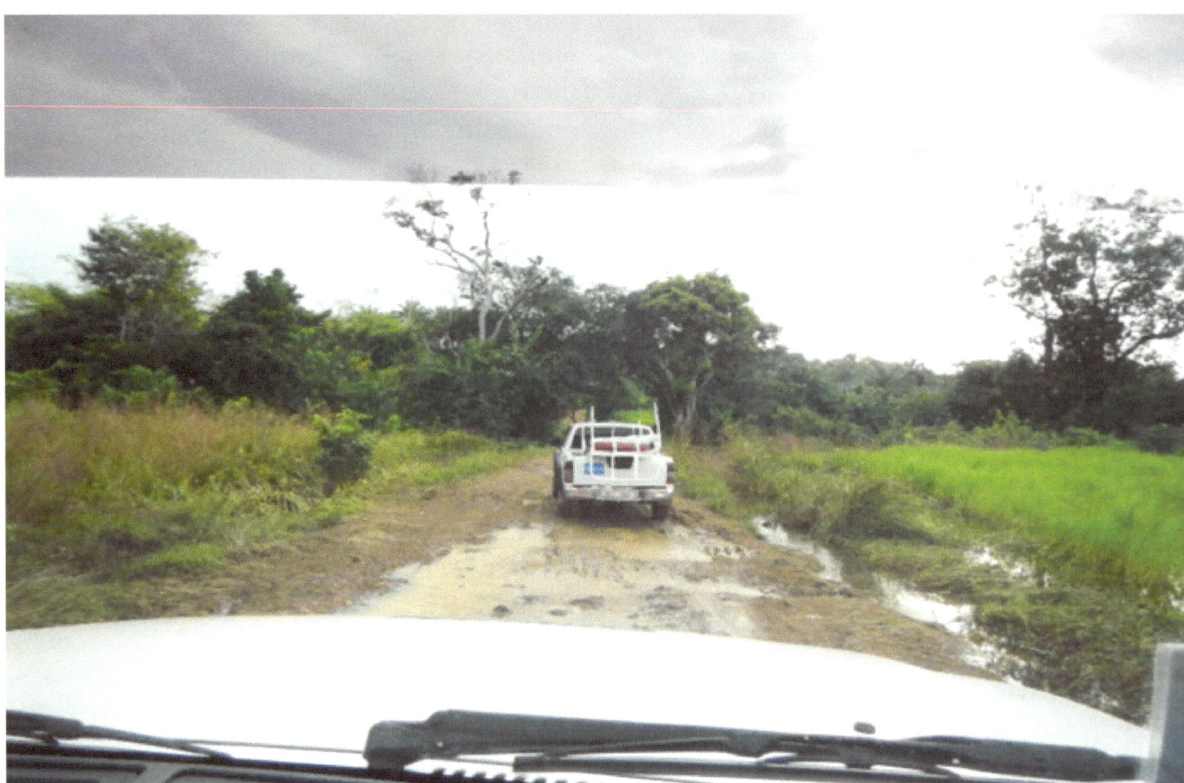

Supplies being delivered to remote areas.

CDR Idongesit Essiet-Gibson

"The team was able to leverage the newly established public health infrastructure to address the post-Ebola measles outbreak, further demonstrating its importance."

—Idongesit Essiet-Gibson, PhD, MPH, PMP

CDR Idongesit Essiet-Gibson was part of an agency-based deployment to Liberia. CDR Essiet-Gibson served on the Centers for Disease Control and Prevention (CDC) Epidemiology Team in Montserrado County from April 25 to May 25, 2015. She remembers, "At the time I arrived, the outbreak was already controlled and there were no new cases." CDR Essiet-Gibson's team focused on strengthening the public health infrastructure, which had been established in response to Ebola. The purpose of this effort was to ensure the infrastructure was retained and could be more readily activated in future outbreaks. CDR Essiet-Gibson also participated in the national measles vaccination campaign to address the upsurge in measles cases immediately following the Ebola outbreak. She says, "The team was able to leverage the newly established public health infrastructure to address the post-Ebola measles outbreak, further demonstrating its importance." CDR Essiet-Gibson notes that another valuable experience for the team was the opportunity to support data abstraction and analysis for the Margibi County Ebola Virus Disease (EVD) Knowledge, Attitudes, and Practice study, published in the *Morbidity and Mortality Weekly Report*, July 10, 2015.

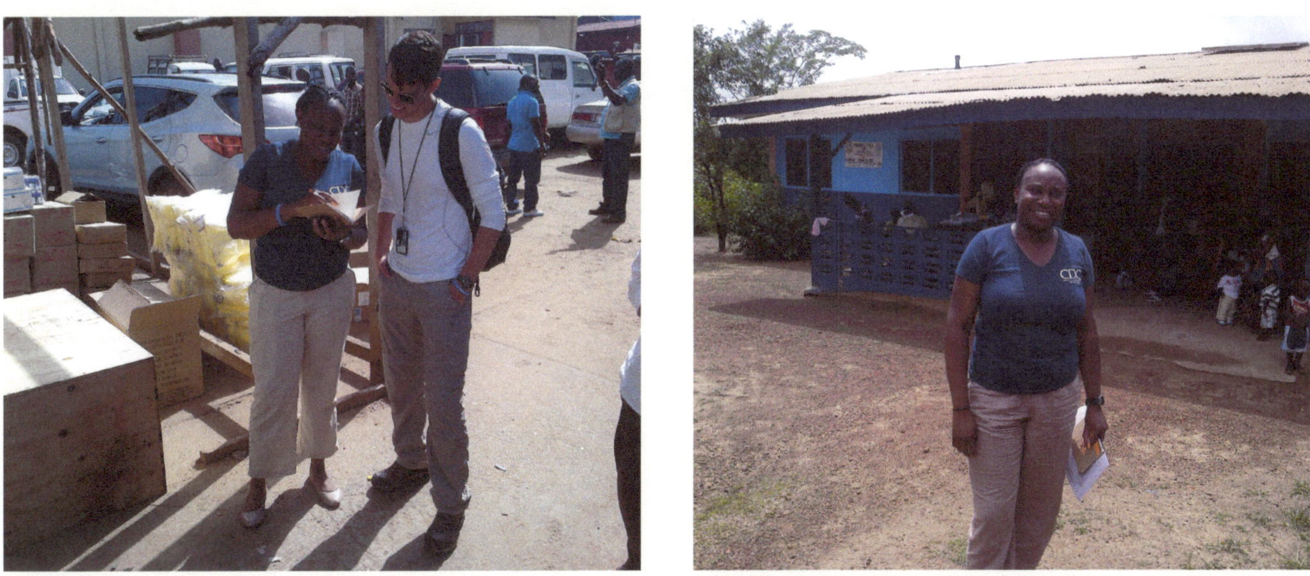

(left) CDR Essiet-Gibson *(left)* takes inventory of measles vaccine supplies outside the Ministry of Health's national measles vaccination distribution warehouse before departing for her daily distributions to supported clinics. *(right)* CDR Essiet-Gibson is shown standing in front of a clinic where she monitored the readiness for the measles vaccination campaign roll-out.

CDR Ibrahim Kamara

"These relationships allowed the Sierra Leone Ministry of Health Division of Surveillance staff to prepare to respond to the Ebola outbreak in densely affected communities with high cases, and as a result, Ebola cases were brought to zero."

—Ibrahim Kamara, MS, MPH, Sc.D.

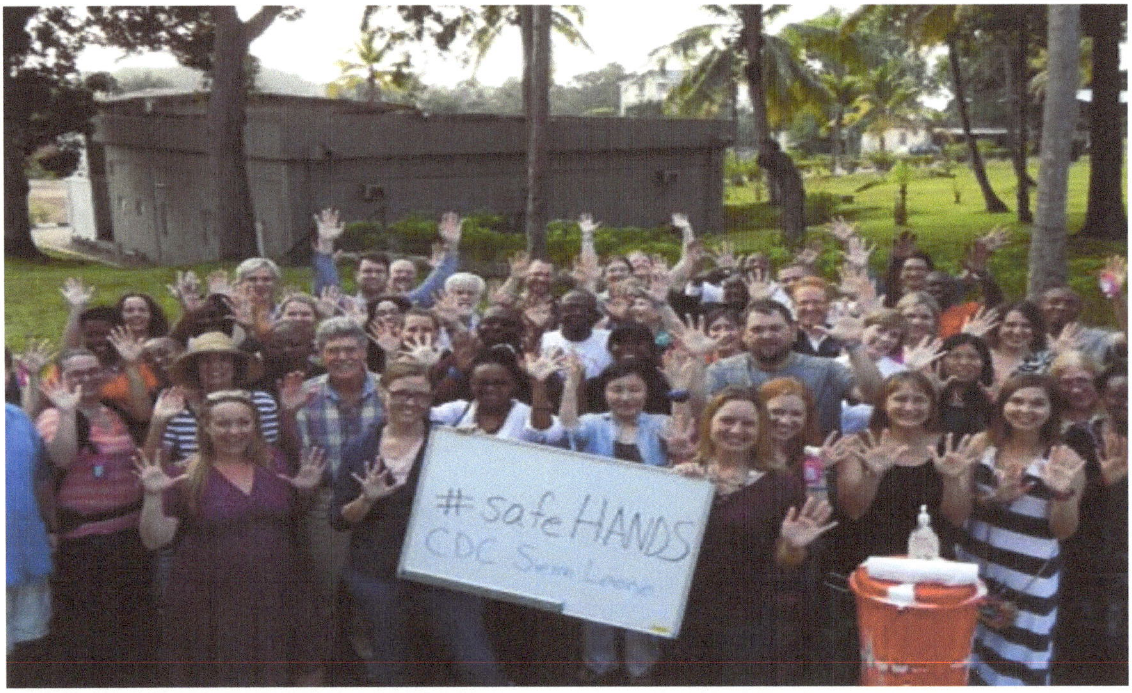

CDR Kamara *(center, directly behind the woman in the front with the white blouse)* with fellow CDC and Corps colleagues in Sierra Leone promoting safe hands practices to prevent the spread of the Ebola virus.

CDR Ibrahim Kamara was deployed with the Centers for Disease Control and Prevention (CDC) Epidemiology Team to Sierra Leone, West Africa, for four months in an attempt to reduce the Ebola prevalence to zero. He designed and presented basic refresher training courses in epidemiology, contact tracing, data analysis, and interpretation of laboratory reports to US government and CDC partners such as the African Union and World Health Organization (WHO) volunteers, including the district surveillance officers of the Sierra Leone Ministry of Health (MOH). In addition, CDR Kamara helped to translate messages regarding vaccinations to the local populace using the local dialect. He also explains, "These relationships allowed the Sierra Leone Ministry of Health Division of Surveillance staff to prepare to respond to the Ebola outbreak in densely affected communities with high cases, and as a result, Ebola cases were brought to zero." CDR Kamara also represented the CDC behavioral health component on radio, explaining the CDC initiatives in Krio, the primary dialect spoken in Sierra Leone. He shared says that this effort allowed the "people of Sierra Leone to be informed about risk and benefits of the vaccine trials, which helped reduce barriers in implementing the CDC vaccine initiatives and other CDC programs." He was interviewed twice a week during his time in Africa in the Krio language on the Sierra Leone Broadcasting Station. CDR Kamara's expertise in his field was instrumental in helping to rid the region of Ebola.

CDR Leslie Hausman

"[It] felt as if I had returned home during a difficult time and everyone was working together to accomplish what needed to be done. . . ."

—Leslie Hausman MPH, BSN, RN

CDR Leslie Hausman deployed twice to the response. In her first deployment, she served on the Ebola Health Promotion/Health Communications Team in Sierra Leone, West Africa, from September 4 to October 2, 2014. CDR Hausman served as a Centers for Disease Control and Prevention (CDC) representative on Sierra Leone's Ebola Social Mobilization Pillar and Messaging Committee. She identified, developed, and supported national Ebola health education and communication and provided feedback to artists on national media campaigns, such as jingles, songs, videos, and posters. She collaborated with non-governmental organizations (NGOs) studying public knowledge, attitudes, and practices related to Ebola prevention and medical care in Sierra Leone. She engaged with in-country CDC staff and partners to support national, district-level, and community-level Ebola-related health information and health promotion needs, and she collaborated with key players, including the World Health Organization (WHO), the United Nations Children's Fund, and the Ministry of Health (MOH). CDR Hausman also collaborated with the US Embassy's Public Affairs Office, disseminating the CDC's Ebola's critical messaging. She subsequently deployed as a Border Health Team lead to Sierra Leone from December 1, 2015, to February 3, 2016. In this role, she collaborated with the CDC and interagency partners working at the airport and seaports in Freetown and both official and unofficial land border crossings between Kambia, Sierra Leone, and Forecariah, Guinea. CDR Hausman provided technical support to the International Organization for Migration, the Ministry of Health and Sanitation, the Sierra Leone Civil Aviation Authority, the Sierra Leone Port Authority, and other response partners concerning the Ebola outbreak, epidemic prone diseases, public health preparedness, cross-border surveillance, and epidemiology. She also assisted with the planning for capacity building for Port Health and Ministry of Health and Sanitation staff during the transition from active response mode to routine operations, including cross-border and port-of-entry surveillance. CDR Hausman recalls, "The impact that serving in this response had on me was immeasurable. I served as a Peace Corps volunteer in Sierra Leone, and it was an honor retuning in a response capacity to the country I view as a second home. Partnering with our Sierra Leone counterparts, transferring sustainable skills, and building public health capacity felt as if I had returned home during a difficult time and everyone was working together to accomplish what needed to be done to stop the transmission of Ebola Virus Disease (EVD) and keep the community healthy and safe."

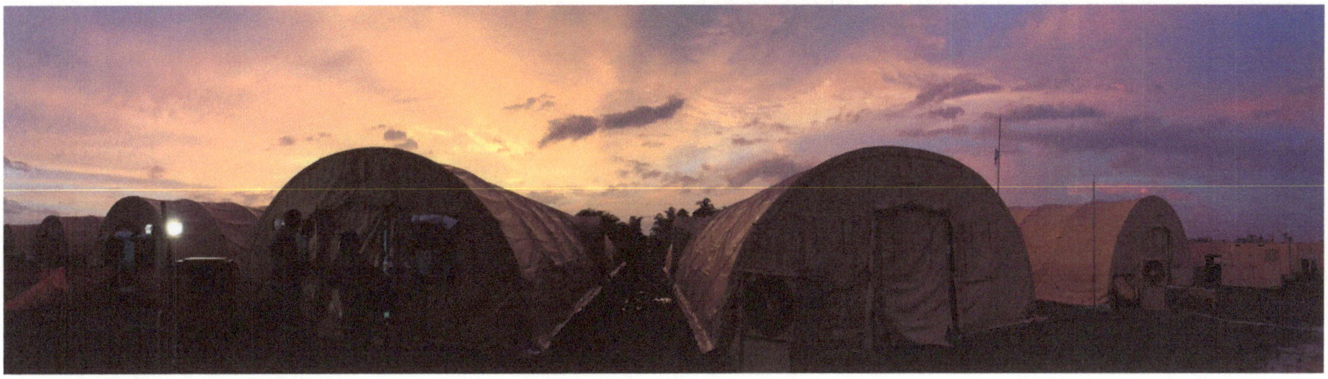

The sun rises over Camp Eason.

CDR Carolina Luna-Pinto

"This was the first time I had seen an entire community affected by a devastating disease."

—Carolina Luna-Pinto, MPH, CHES

CDR Carolina Luna-Pinto deployed both internationally and domestically to support the Ebola response. While in Liberia, she led the Border Health Team in building capacity among port workers at airports, seaports, and land border crossings to support exit screening and response efforts through technical assistance, training, and outreach. In the US, CDR Luna-Pinto was key early in the development of training materials that were initially adapted to prepare port workers in Liberia, Guinea, Sierra Leone, Mali, and Senegal for exit screening. These materials were used in preparedness efforts in countries not affected by Ebola, which led to the adaptation of the RING tool (Recognize, Isolate, Notify, Give Support) as a way to introduce response efforts at ports of entry and the development of posters describing personal protective equipment (PPE) guidance for port workers based on their role.

CDR Luna-Pinto deployed for forty days to support entry screening efforts at the Centers for Disease Control and Prevention (CDC) Washington, DC, Quarantine Station to improve procedures for their Check and Report Ebola (CARE) Ambassadors program and implement changes to the entry-screening process. CDR Luna-Pinto recalls,

"This was the first time I had seen an entire community affected by a devastating disease. Every person had been touched in one way or another by the disease and had family that had lost their lives to the disease. No longer were we dealing with a disease that could spread; it had already spread and was affecting the livelihood of Liberia. Being able to work side by side with Liberians to train as many people on how to protect themselves, their families, and their communities was critical."

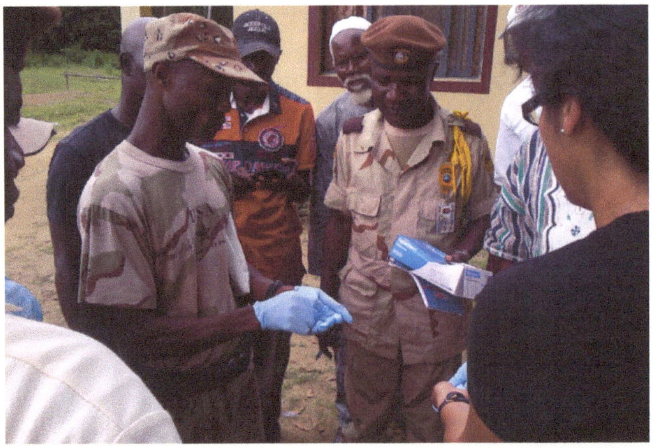

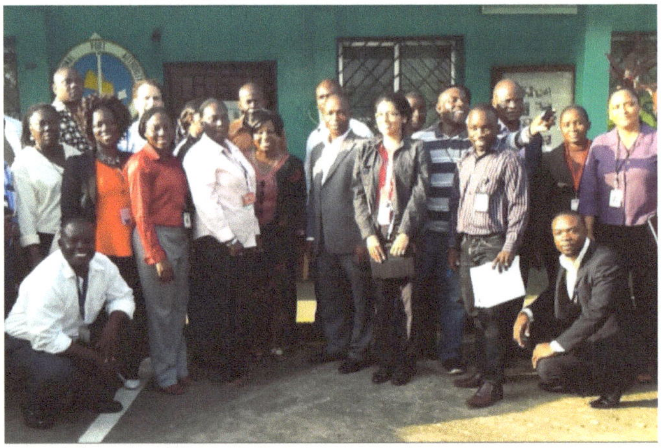

(left) CDR Luna-Pinto on the border of Liberia and Sierra Leone delivering just-in-time training to border patrol agents and border town members, including the chief, on PPE. This photo shows the proper removal of gloves. *(right)* CDR Luna-Pinto *(front right of center)* is seen here with port-of-entry stakeholders after delivering a two-day Train-the-Trainer course on Ebola prevention strategies.

CDR Erica Sison

"Overall, the Ebola response was both challenging and rewarding. It was over a year of being pushed to our limits."

—Erica Sison, MPH

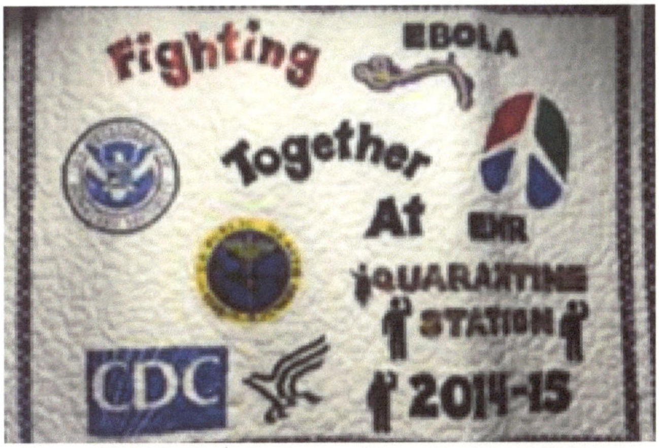

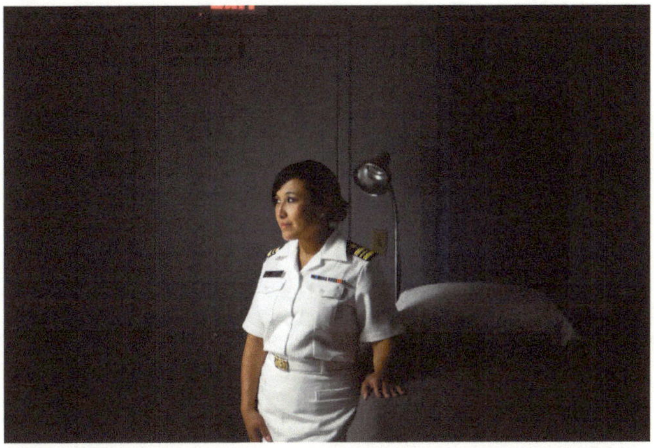

(left) An image of the Fighting Ebola Together sign at Newark Liberty Airport (EWR) Quarantine Station 2014-2015 is displayed. *(right)* An Ebola outbreak in Africa increased the workload for Erica Sison, the head quarantine officer at Newark Liberty Airport.

Adapted from a *New York Times* article (originally published August 8, 2014): During the 2014–2016 Ebola response, CDR Sison led the development, implementation, and management of the Ebola Enhanced Entry Screening (EEES) program at Newark Liberty International Airport as the Officer-in-Charge of the Centers for Disease Control and Prevention (CDC) Newark Quarantine Station. The EEES program was a key component of this multilayered strategy to reduce the likelihood of international spread of the virus. In response to the first imported case of Ebola into the United States, the White House National Security Council gave a directive to initiate the EEES. In October 2014, EEES was established exclusively at five US airports to identify travelers arriving via airports, seaports, and land borders from countries with widespread Ebola transmission. These five airports accounted for 94 percent of all travelers into the United States from affected countries. EEES ended in February 2016. In her own words, CDR Sison recounts, "Overall, the Ebola response was both challenging and rewarding. It was over a year of being pushed to our limits. Often, in times of stress, we can make it or break it, but all the people that were here to support the mission were the best of the best. They made this all happen and did it with a great attitude throughout the process. We were nothing without this team who turned into our family. Sometimes there were growing pains, but we worked through them together. We were lucky to have met so many phenomenal people and learn so much about all the tremendous public health work and impact each was making in the world. What truly felt like teamwork was so many people coming from different agencies and backgrounds to accomplish one goal and mission. Each responder was ready from day one to fulfill the daily tasks and to support each other. No one was above any task, no matter how tedious. We were most happy for West Africa for their success of controlling the outbreak. Our hearts and prayers were continuously with them while they lived through the outbreak and as they recovered."

LCDR Sylvera Demas

"In Guinea, I was able to see that my contribution, like many others, made a big difference..."

—Sylvera Demas, MPH, CPH

LCDR Sylvera Demas was involved in the 2014–2015 Ebola response, deploying three times and each time playing a different role. First, he deployed to the Centers for Disease Control and Prevention (CDC) Emergency Operations Center from October 27 to November 26, 2014, where he assisted with the development and the implementation of the CDC employee monitoring program. He recalls, "There I developed messages and contacted returned deployers from West Africa to inform them of and enroll them in the program. I also followed up with them until their twenty-one days of monitoring were over." LCDR Demas collected important information to share with agency leadership, which ultimately led to the CDC administrative leave for deployers, a letter sent to deployers signed by the CDC director to show that they have completed their twenty-one days of monitoring and were not a threat to the public. In LCDR Demas's second deployment, he was sent to Guinea. From January 14 to February 12, 2015, he served as a public health advisor with the CDC's Division of Global Migration and Quarantine. About this role, LCDR Demas shares, "I provided technical assistance and made recommendations to Guinea Ministry of Health (MOH) and Ministry of Transportation (MOT) on border-health issues, monitored entry and exit screenings of passengers at Conakry Airport, and assisted the MOH and MOT in developing maritime Standard Operating Procedures to be implemented through all Guinea sea ports." In addition, LCDR Demas wrote proposals to the CDC Foundation requesting funds for Ebola response activities at sea ports and Conakry Airport. On a subsequent deployment to Guinea the following year from January 18 to February 28, 2016, he served as the Ebola response deputy for Guinea. He provided coordination and management of all activities for the CDC Guinea Ebola Response Team, conducted orientation for all staff deployed to Guinea, and coordinated with the World Health Organization (WHO) for staff to attend WHO security briefings. Importantly, LCDR Demas contributed to presentations to brief the CDC director and participated in conference calls to update him regarding the Ebola response activities and challenges in Guinea. Likewise, he prepared weekly bullets to update CDC headquarters on the activities and challenges of Guinea team. LCDR Demas shares, "In Guinea, I was able to see that my contribution, like many others, made a big difference because during my second deployment, Guinea reached 'Zero Ebola.' Schools were opened, constructions workers returned to work, and businesses re-opened."

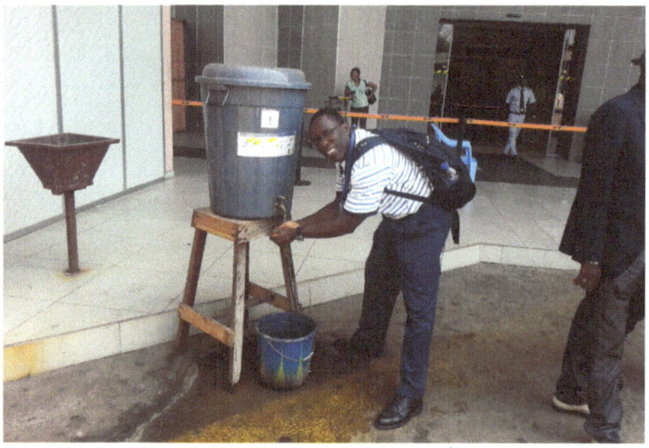

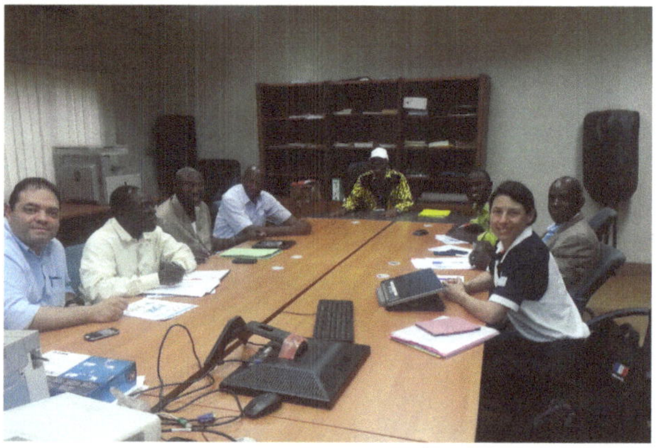

(left) LCDR Sylvera Demas washes his hands with chlorinated water at the handwashing station before entering the "Controle Sanitaire," where passengers were screened before checking in at the Conakry Airport. *(right)* LCDR Sylvera Demas *(second on the left)* and his teammate, Joaquin Rueda, attend an Aviation Civile weekly planning meeting, which was held every Wednesday at the Direction Nationale de l'Aviation Civile building in Conakry, Guinea.

LCDR Arthur Hurst

"It was a reminder of the true value of our mission, not only protecting global health, but also in improving the lives of individuals."

—Arthur Hurst, MS

LCDR Arthur Hurst deployed with the Centers for Disease Control and Prevention (CDC) to Port Loko, Sierra Leone, from September 3 through October 15, 2015. LCDR Hurst was part of the Sierra Leone Trial to Introduce a Vaccine against Ebola (STRIVE), a phase II/III trial that was designed to assess the safety and efficacy of the rVSV-ZEBOV candidate Ebola vaccine. During the deployment, LCDR Hurst served as the STRIVE Port Loko Lead and worked with the local vaccine-trial partners in the Port Loko district. He assisted local partners with logistics, communication, and operational challenges involved in the vaccine trial, including vaccination and data management activities. LCDR Hurst remembers the genuine gratitude that the Sierra Leone people had toward the CDC personnel: "It made a huge impression on me. Even strangers on the street would thank me for my work. It was a reminder of the true value of our mission, not only protecting global health, but also in improving the lives of individuals."

LT Allen Applegate

"Going back to basics—seeing the real impact of implementing basic public health measures, such as basic hand hygiene—can have huge impact."

—Allen Applegate, DrPH, MPH, CPH

LT Allen Applegate deployed to Monrovia, Liberia, from June 10 to July 13, 2015. During his time in Liberia, LT Applegate served as the Border Health Team lead, where his focus was to prevent or mitigate the importation or exportation of Ebola to other countries, including the US, in compliance with International Health Regulations. In this role, he had many responsibilities, including coordinating with border partners, such as the Ministry of Health (MOH), the World Health Organization (WHO), and the International Organization for Migration and Global Communities, to build additional surveillance capacity through the development of the Integrated Disease Surveillance and Response framework for border health. LT Applegate recalls, "New clusters of Ebola cases near Roberts International Airport in the summer of 2015 presented a number of challenges. Our team had to quickly shift priorities to coordinate daily with port partners to ensure passenger manifests were checked against lists of contacts indented." Additionally, when faced with potential workforce shortages, LT Applegate and his team quickly developed and provided just-in-time training to develop additional screening capacity for port health workers on recognizing signs and symptoms of Ebola, passenger exit screening process, basic hand hygiene, and personal protective equipment (PPE). Of his experiences, LT Applegates shares "Going back to basics—seeing the real impact of implementing basic public health measures, such as basic hand hygiene—can have huge impact."

LT Jennifer Johnson

"I'm proud and honored to have played a small role in this effort."

—Jennifer Johnson MPH

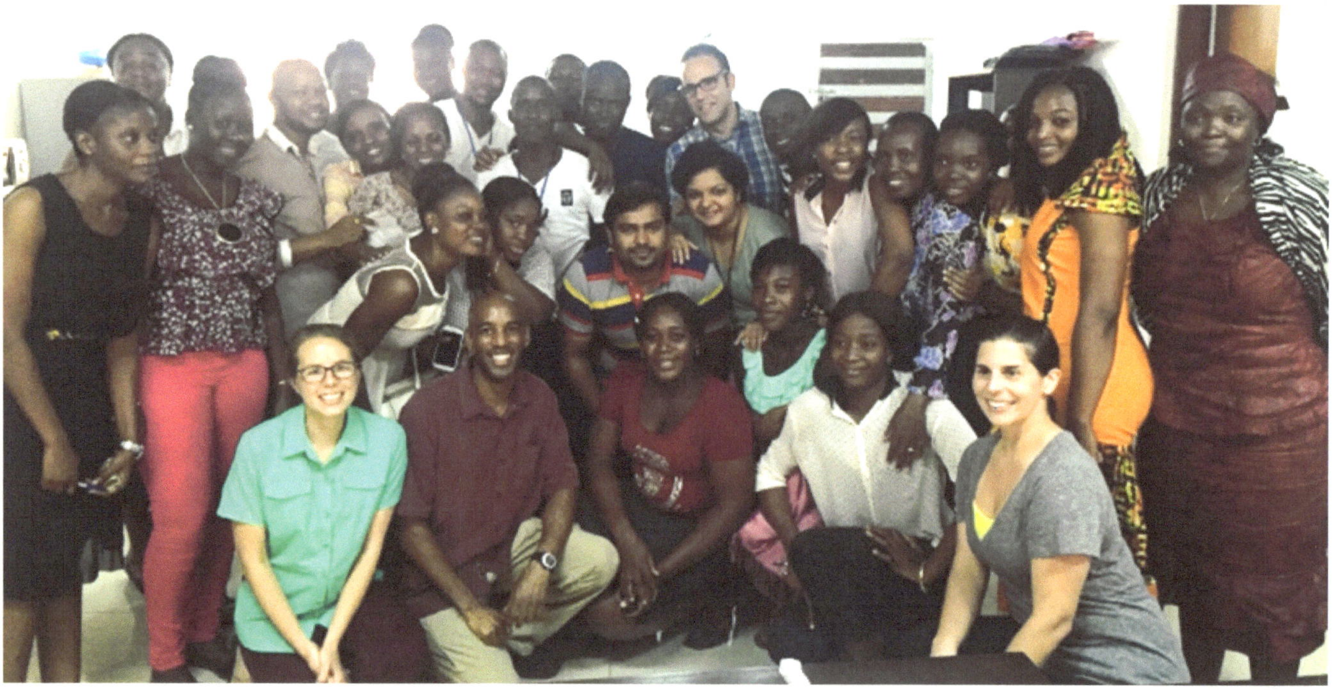

The Data Center team celebrates a milestone in STRIVE study progress. The people working at this Data Center were dedicated to following up with study subjects to collect data on safety and effectiveness.

LT Jennifer Johnson deployed with the USPHS Commissioned Corps to assist with the Sierra Leone Trial to Introduce a Vaccine against Ebola (STRIVE). LT Johnson worked at a data center in Freetown, providing support to the team responsible for collecting safety and efficacy data on subjects who had received the vaccine. LT Johnson recalls,

"There are so many challenges to implementing a clinical trial during an ongoing outbreak in a resource-poor country like Sierra Leone. Everything from road infrastructure to internet connectivity to safety concerns made this environment different from any clinical trial I have ever seen. And yet, this was the only place where the trial could be. The perseverance of those involved in STRIVE to keep going despite these challenges impressed upon me the shared sense of purpose and importance of our work. I'm proud and honored to have played a small role in this effort."

LT Samantha Morgan

"It was incredible to see how little physical resources these village towns had, yet the people of the village went above and beyond to help however they could."

—Samantha Morgan, MPH

LT Samantha Morgan was deployed to Senegal, West Africa, from February 7 to March 11, 2015. LT Morgan assisted with the Ebola response as part of the High-Risk Unaffected Countries Team. She conducted a border assessment with international partners (the World Health Organization (WHO), the US Agency for International Development, the United Nations (UN) International Children's Emergency Fund, and International Organization of Migration) and developed recommendations for the Ministry of Health (MOH) to fundamentally change the screening process of individuals entering the country. LT Morgan recounts,

"It was incredible to see how little physical resources these village towns had, yet the people of the village went above and beyond to help however they could. **All of the village men volunteered to staff a handwashing station around the clock, twenty-four seven, in an effort to protect their village. It was a very humbling experience that I'll never forget."**

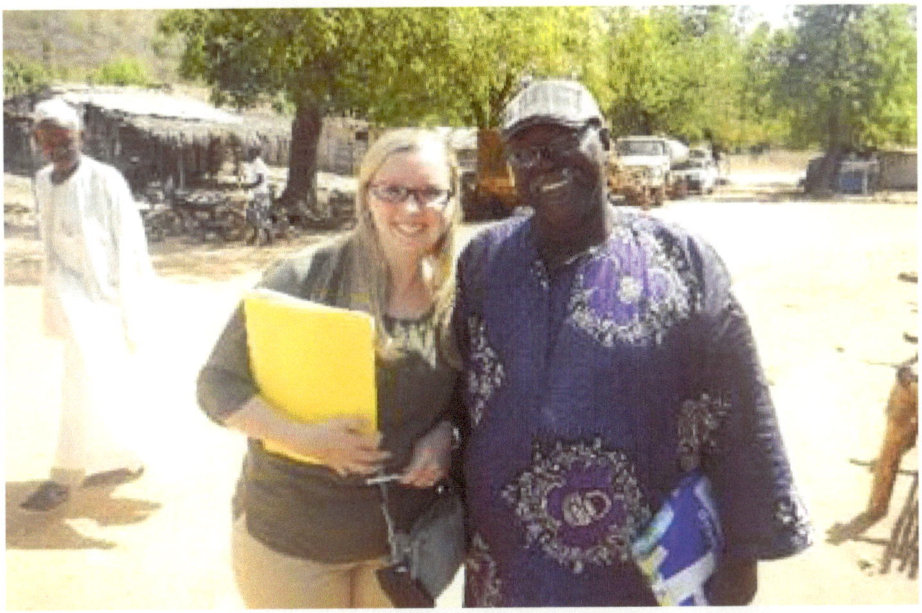

LT Morgan *(left)* and the single nurse at the border station. The male nurse was the only medical personnel within a thirty-minute drive from the border station.

LT Janesia Robbs

"[I had to] assure the gentleman that the work he did not have a chance to complete was not in vain. I helped lift his spirit to see the larger impact of the work he had done and would continue to do on the mainland."

—Janesia Robbs, MPH, MCHES

LT Janesia Robbs was deployed from December 22, 2014, through January 21, 2015, as a Check and Report Ebola (CARE) ambassador to the Centers for Disease Control and Prevention (CDC) Atlanta Quarantine Station. In that role, LT Robbs was responsible for providing Ebola-related information to travelers arriving in the US from Guinea, Liberia, and Sierra Leone. During her time at the Atlanta Quarantine Station, LT Robbs participated in a three-day CARE ambassador training session and ultimately provided over fifty CARE encounters with travelers. Following her deployment, LT Robbs was invited to travel back to Atlanta to support entry screening efforts for the return of USPHS Commissioned Corps officers assigned to the Monrovia Medical Unit (MMU) Team 2 returning from Liberia. LT Robbs is proud to report the team expeditiously screened all seventy-two officers and prepared them for twenty-one days of active monitoring.

Through this deployment, LT Robbs had an opportunity to use her health education skills and background to protect and promote public health in the US and meet a diverse, dedicated, and passionate group of CDC workers. One of the best experiences that LT Robbs had on this mission was greeting a very unhappy and despairing CDC worker who was returning from Guinea. She states, "I had to put on my brightest smile, which I am known for, and assure the gentleman that the work he did not have a chance to complete was not in vain. I helped lift his spirit to see the larger impact of the work he had done and would continue to do on the mainland."

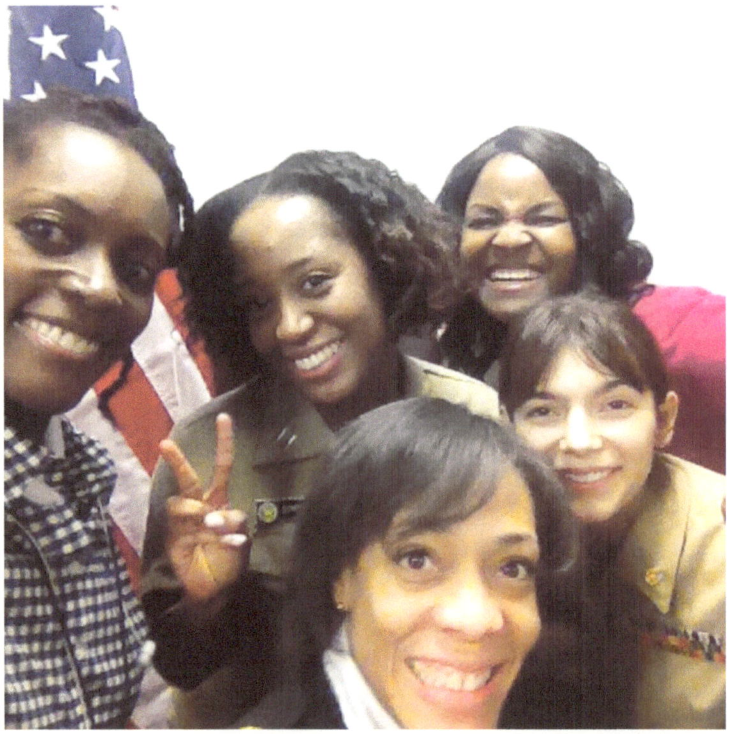

LT Robbs *(featured center)* pose-s with the team at the CDC Quarantine Station.

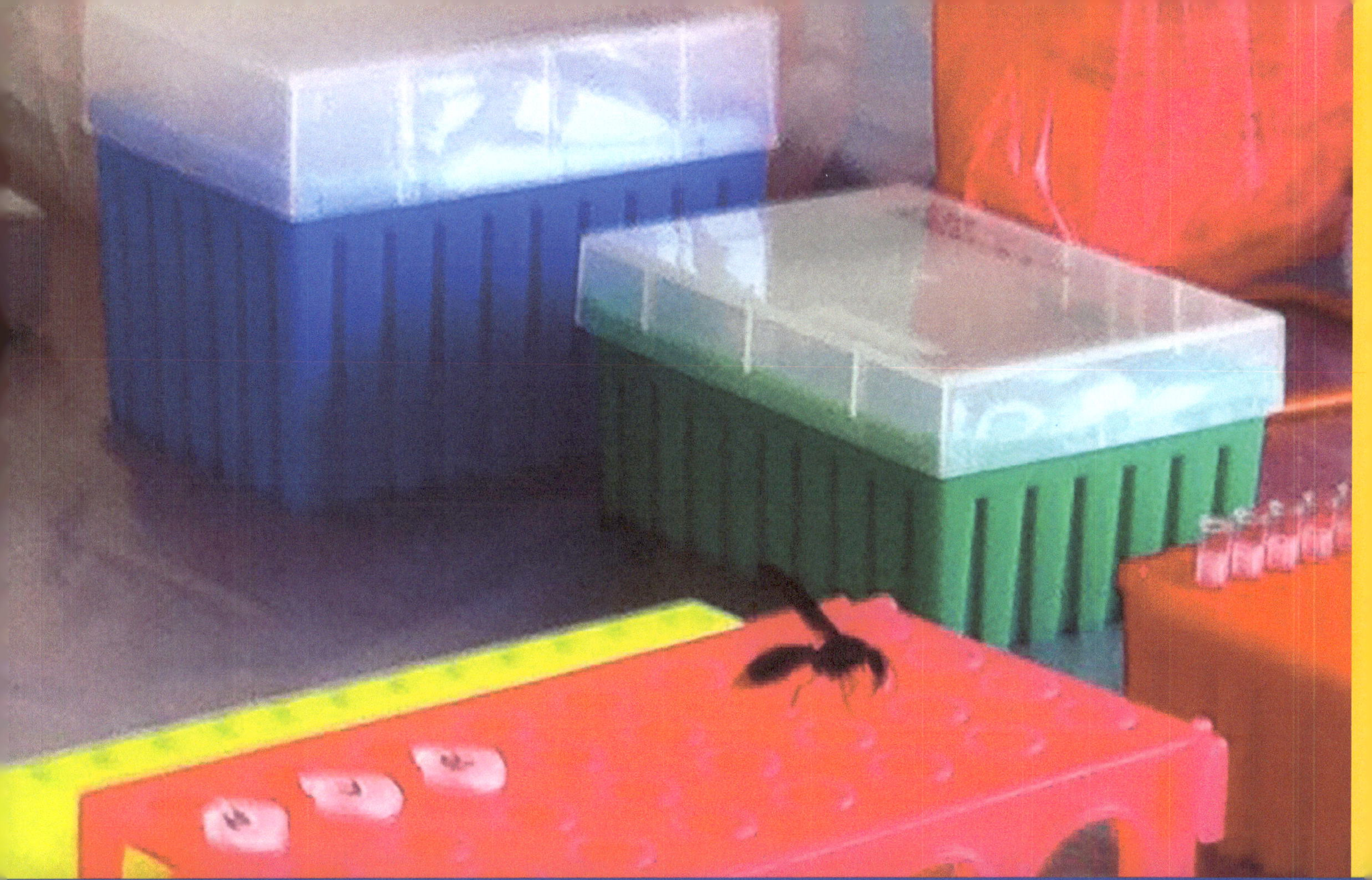

DETECT

"Detection is the 'revelation of what is concealed' (Merriam-Webster Dictionary). Health services officers working to detect Ebola Virus Disease (EVD) served in a myriad of environs from makeshift testing laboratories in the jungles of the African continent, to border security checkpoints along remote dusty roads, to United States international airports. These officers were involved in epidemiology, surveillance, contact tracing, border health screening, laboratory testing, and research. Officers brought their extensive training and expertise to bear on rapid detection of infection and subsequent contact tracing to contain the spread of Ebola virus."

Jessica Damon, MPH, MLS
CDR, USPHS

Detection of disease is the second pillar in the Global Health Security framework and can be described as the ability to identify an infectious disease that has the potential to be a significant threat to the health and safety of nations. Primary detection begins at the individual level and includes the ability to identify and diagnose disease causing agents accurately and efficiently. Once identified, the capacity to monitor disease incidence at the community level and to track disease movement within and beyond local boundaries, forms the subsequent layer of disease detection efforts. This layer requires protocols and systems both physical and technological to support widespread surveillance efforts. Activities that support detection efforts involve laboratory testing, disease reporting, epidemiological tracking, border control and research to better predict disease movement through populations. As with the previous section, the stories in the section are introduced by the 2014 HSPAC Chair, CAPT Todd Alspach who provides perspective as the response unfolds. It also features a Force Leadership Highlight by LCDR Elizabeth Degrange who served as the executive officer to the Incident Commander providing a vital link to response planning and preparation. These two features are intended to set the stage for the stories that follow. The officer accounts of their work and the impact of participating in these detection efforts are presented following military custom with the highest-ranking officers given the floor first in presentation. Some stories included in the section may have activities that span all three pillars of Global Health Security (prevent, detect, respond) but they have been placed here for the unique examples of the various actions that support disease detection.

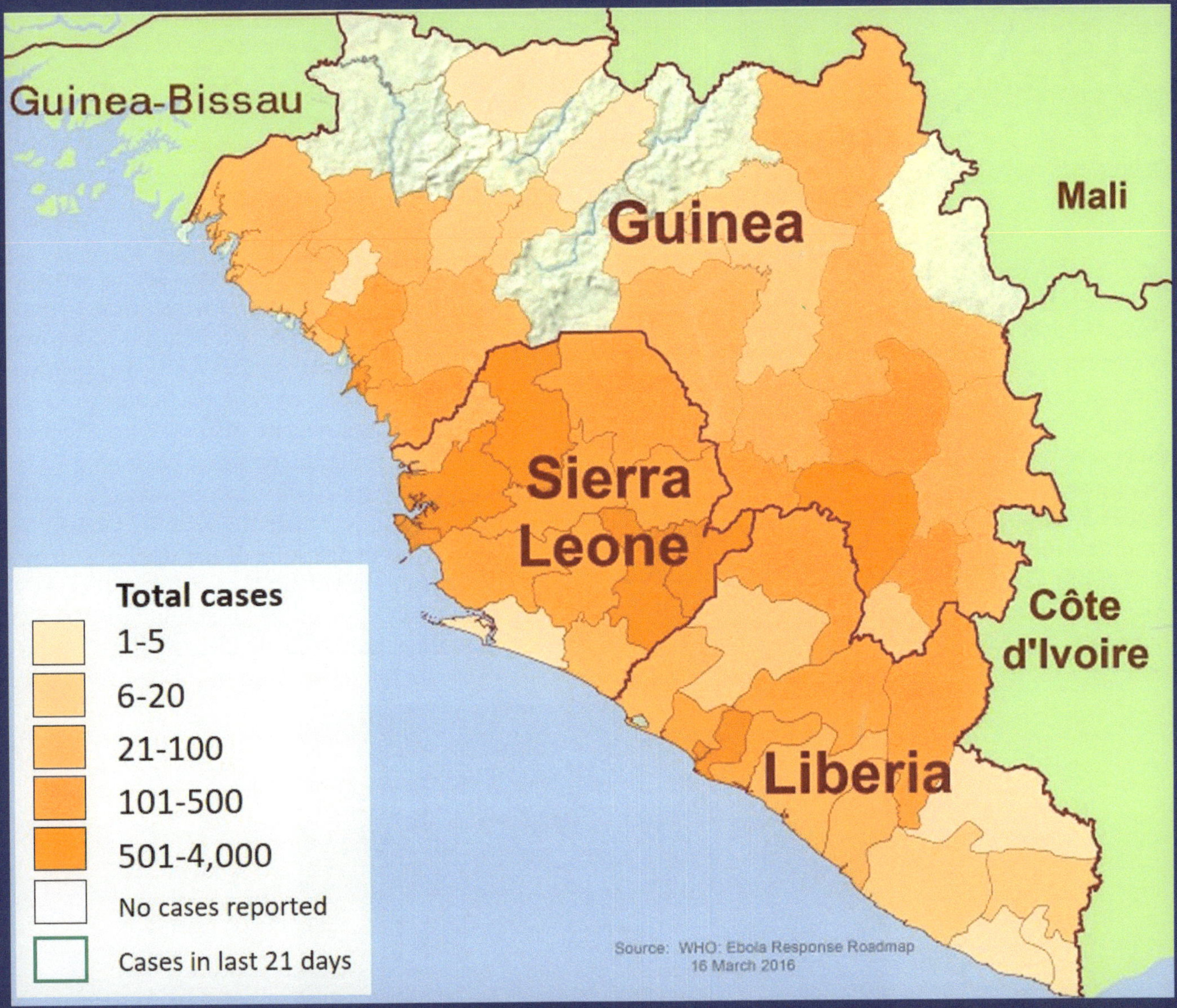

The countries with the most widespread transmission were Guinea, Liberia, and Sierra Leone. A total of 28,616 cases of EVD and 11,310 deaths were reported. There were an additional thirty-six cases and fifteen deaths that occurred when the outbreak spread outside of these three countries.[4]

4—https://www.cdc.gov/vhf/ebola/history/2014-2016-outbreak/index.html

HSPAC CHAIR: Perspective as the Response Begins

CAPT Todd Alspach recalls the start of the Ebola response during the last months of his term as HSPAC Chair: "The Ebola response started at the tail end of 2014. The earliest mention I could find in my notes was from early October 2014. At that point there were only a handful of known health services officers (HSOs) who were tasked with being deployed to West Africa. As a category, we tried to provide as much information as possible with regards to deploying to that particular area. In addition, we disseminated other readiness information related to the deployment, such as two vaccines that were required: typhoid and yellow fever." As the full scale of the epidemic was just beginning to be recognized, CAPT Alspach was preparing to transition the category to its 2015 incumbent chair, CAPT Stacey Evans. CAPT Alspach recalls, "At that point in time, the impact on me as the HSPAC Chair was minimal since it was so late in my term. I thanked the officers deployed in a couple of the weekly blurbs I wrote. But as that mission was really just getting underway, the impact really hadn't been felt yet." CAPT Alspach pointed to the greater impact on CAPT Stacy Evans who was deployed to Liberia in late 2015 at the end of her term in the position. "This meant CDR Bobby Rasulnia, as the Chair Elect in 2015, had to take over in her absence."

> **"As a category, we tried to provide as much information as possible with regards to deploying to that particular area."**
>
> *—Todd Alspach, MOS, CLC (AMT), MT (ASCP), CAPT, USPHS*
> Health Services Professional Advisory Committee (HSPAC) Chair, 2014

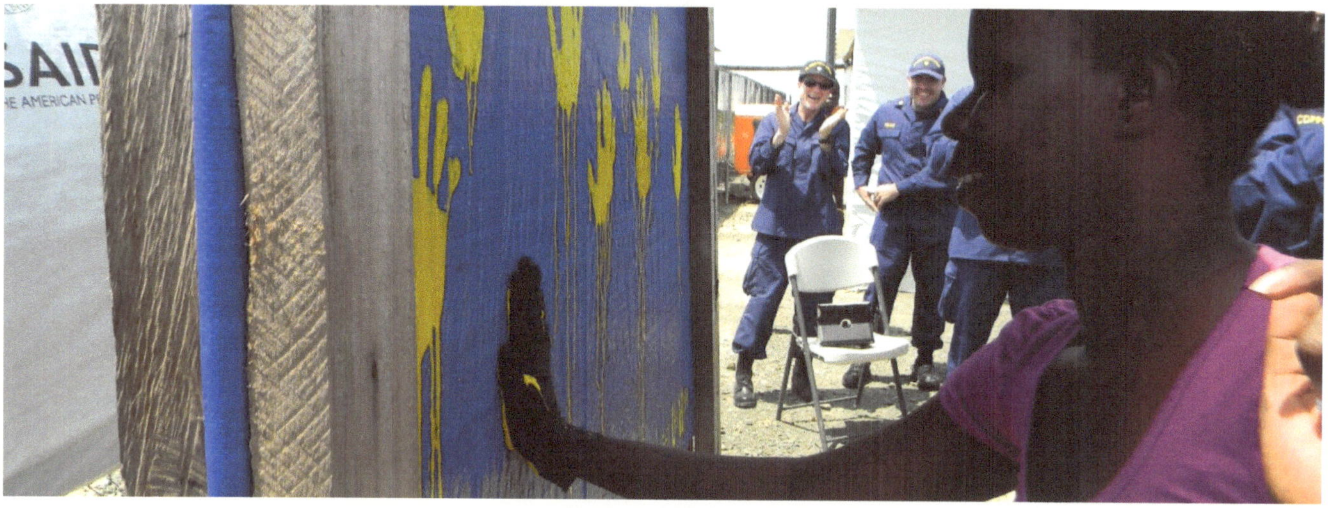

A Liberian Ebola patient of the MMU places her hand dipped in yellow paint on the historic MMU Survivor Wall.

Todd Alspach, MOS, CLC (AMT), MT (ASCP)

CAPT, USPHS

HSPAC Chair, 2015

CAPT Todd Alspach is a certified medical technologist with a master's degree in occupational health and safety. He is currently assigned to the Centers for Medicare and Medicaid Services as the regional laboratory consultant in Denver, Colorado. CAPT Alspach previously served with the Food and Drug Administration (FDA), the Federal Bureau of Prisons (BOP), and the Centers for Disease Control and Prevention (CDC) during his sixteen-year career with the United States Public Health Service (USPHS). He is an active member of the Health Services category, where he was appointed to two terms on the HSPAC as a voting member and served as the 2014 HSPAC Chair. He currently serves as deputy commander of Regional Incident Support Team 8 and is a highly committed mentor to numerous officers.

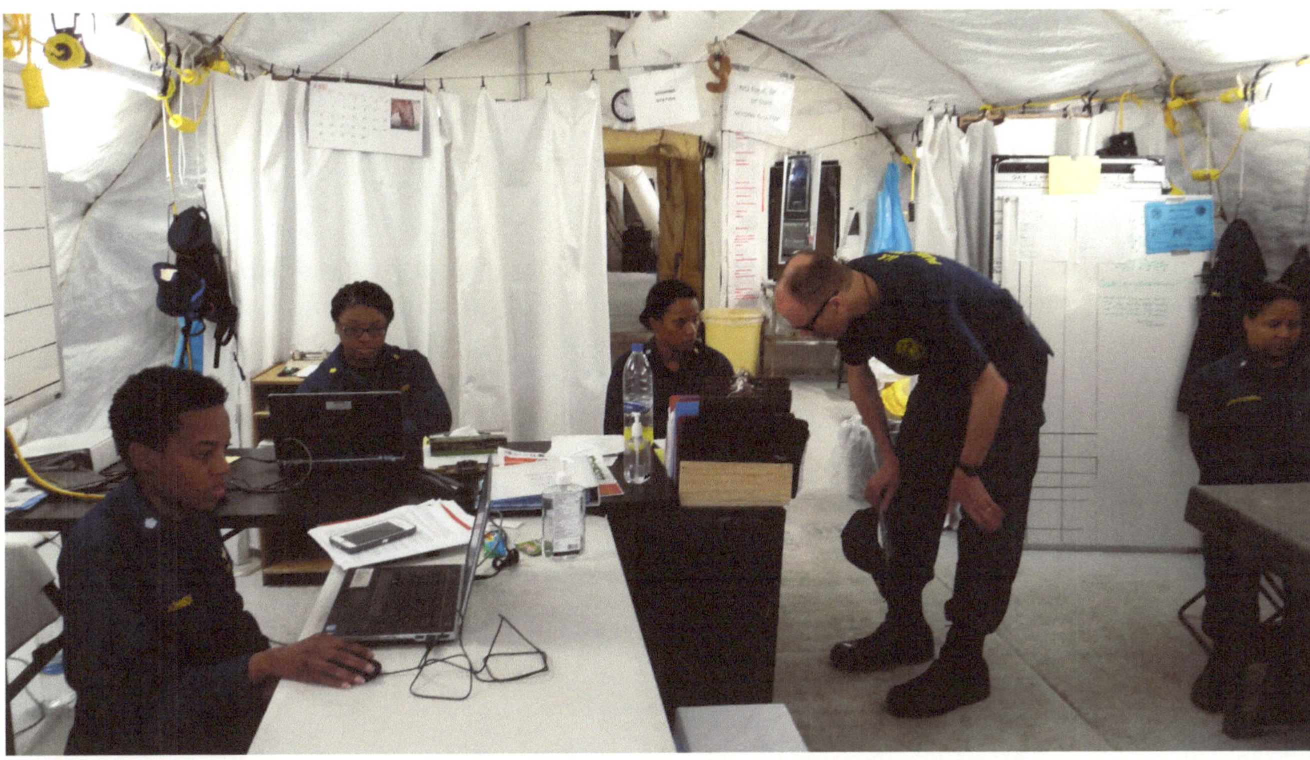

Daily life at the Monrovia Medical Unit (MMU), showing officers in action at the command and control center.

Force Leadership Highlight

LCDR Elizabeth DeGrange

"The willingness of people to serve in so many unknown and dangerous situations . . . was impressive."

—Elizabeth DeGrange, MS, MFS

LCDR Elizabeth DeGrange served as the training coordinator for the Readiness and Deployment Operations Group (RedDOG). At the time of the outbreak she was third in command for overseeing the Commissioned Corps Ebola response, serving as the training officer, logistics officer, and travel officer, while RADM Scott Giberson served as the Ebola incident commander with CAPT Dan Beck as the deputy incident commander. In addition, LCDR DeGrange deployed with Monrovia Medical Unit (MMU) Team 4 for thirty-eight days and served as the executive officer for RADM Giberson, conducting front-end planning for US Surgeon General VADM Vivek Murthy's 2015 visit. LCDR DeGrange recalls the impact of the officer response to the early call for volunteers to deploy: "We sent this request out across September 13–14, 2014, and by September 17, we had 5,160 responses! Although not all officers had approved availability, 4,300 respondents, including retirees, were ready to go to West Africa in support of the Ebola response, even without knowing a lot of the details. We asked officers to fill these various roles: support clinical care, behavioral health, public health education, administration, logistics, liaison, as well as command and control. This really stood out for me. Through the entirety of the mission, the willingness of people to serve in so many unknown and dangerous situations and get to know the community was impressive."

"Looking back four years now, I have seen the positive impact it has had across the Corps. It helped create a culture that is more focused on being prepared for deployment. It resulted in motivating officers to be fit and meet basic readiness requirements. It promoted a greater appreciation for deployment roles and responsibilities." LCDR DeGrange recalls that some officers who volunteered to deploy were listed as ineligible due to a failure to maintain all readiness requirements, and that this left a deep impression on officers of the importance of being basic ready and documenting their clinical skills. Another positive outgrowth of this response was a Corps commitment to being more intentional in taking care of deployed and returning officers and their families. The Family Support Network (FSN) was instrumental in creating support for officers and their families over the course of the response and aided in the recommendation for, and creation of what is now, the Corps

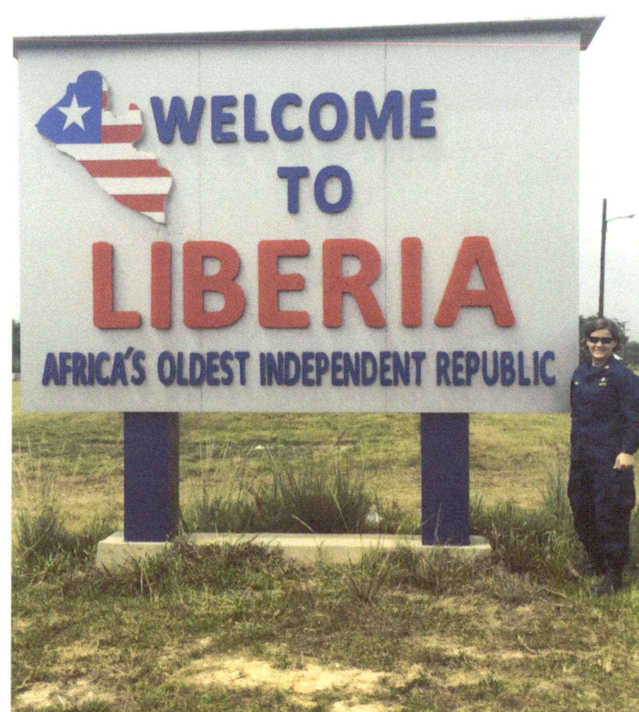

LCDR DeGrange arrives in Liberia.

Care program. "The mission resulted in so many positive changes in how officers viewed response and mission impact."

LCDR DeGrange shared that many officers were deeply moved by the simple, inherent value of the buddy system: each officer was paired with a "battle buddy" and charged with watching out and caring for that other officer in a mutually supportive way. This ensured that they each reached the end of the mission safely. Although it has been several years since the response, many of the battle buddies (and entire MMU teams) from this response stay in very close contact. The friendships made were deep, abiding, and genuine. The impacts were also positive among leaders, particularly in the Office of the Assistant Secretary for Preparedness and Response, and have had a direct influence on recent hurricane missions. For these missions, behavioral health assets were integrated into the deployment teams as well as into the Incident Management Team to support officers throughout the deployment experience. These individuals welcomed officers home with words of thanks and support, simple signs, and food. This type of response was learned through the success of the Ebola response model, and it had a rewarding and long-lasting mental health impact on responders.

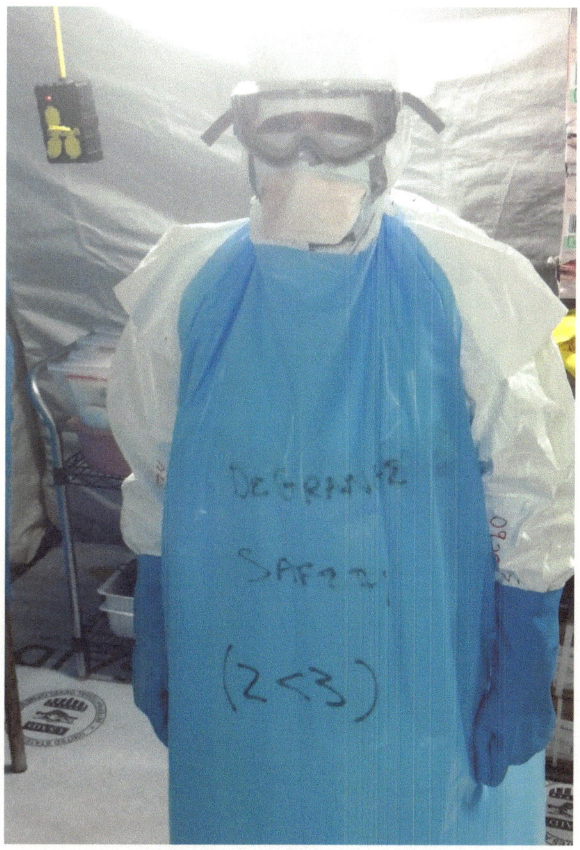

LCDR DeGrange peers out from behind her googles, dressed out in full personal protective equipment (PPE).

"For me, it was awesome to be part of the operational team. In theater there was a ton of support from the Department of Defense (DOD), who even made sure the Corps had an office at the old Embassy alongside them. Médecins Sans Frontières (MSF), both in Anniston and in theater, made for valuable and experienced partners. The Disaster Assistance Response Team (DART) was awesome. Their willingness to share information and work together created such a collegial atmosphere." LCDR DeGrange recalled that she was honored to work with and have the support of Assistant Secretary for Health Karen DeSalvo, US Surgeon General Vivek Murthy, and Deputy US Surgeon General RADM Boris Lushniak. Our senior leadership developed strong partnerships with MSF and DART as well as the Center for Domestic Preparedness (CDP). Being able to partner with MSF was hugely beneficial, especially when developing the Ebola Treatment Unit (ETU) Training at CDP. We were able to incorporate their experience managing ETUs into the training our officers would receive. "Being a health services officer (HSO) made it much easier for me," recalls DeGrange, "because I know these positions and functions required to make a large-scale deployment like our Ebola response run, and I intimately know what the Health Services category brings to the table for the Corps." LCDR DeGrange worked with the chief professional officers (CPOs) to do officer skill and readiness checks, identifying officers that would make a robustly skilled team. These names were then sent to agency liaisons. As needed, CPOs continued to make additional recommendations to fit for specific positions needs.

LCDR DeGrange was complimentary of her predecessor's leadership and foresight. She said, "RADM Elizondo did some great work there, and it was amazing for me to be able to see it through. For example, he had worked to organize a summit of local leaders and educators, desiring to put them all in the same room to talk about the disease and their experience. He left before this could take place, and it was really cool for me to ensure that his vision was carried out, and a very special event to be a part of." The panel discussion took place at Monrovia City Hall a few weeks after his departure and one of the many topics discussed was how to rebuild sustainable health systems.

LCDR DeGrange explained,

> "Health services officers strongly impacted the success of this mission. It was this category that developed and executed a cross-disciplinary train-the-trainer workshop in which other healthcare workers from outside ETUs, came to the MMU and trained with the Corps. Subsequently, MMU Corps officers also went to their ETUs and trained on site with them. Training was provided in everything from hand washing to the use of ultrasound to performance of CPR to resiliency. It was a four-day workshop for all healthcare workers and resulted in a certificate of completion with a graduation. It is the multidisciplinary nature of this category that lends us to be successful with a lot of the developing mission needs."

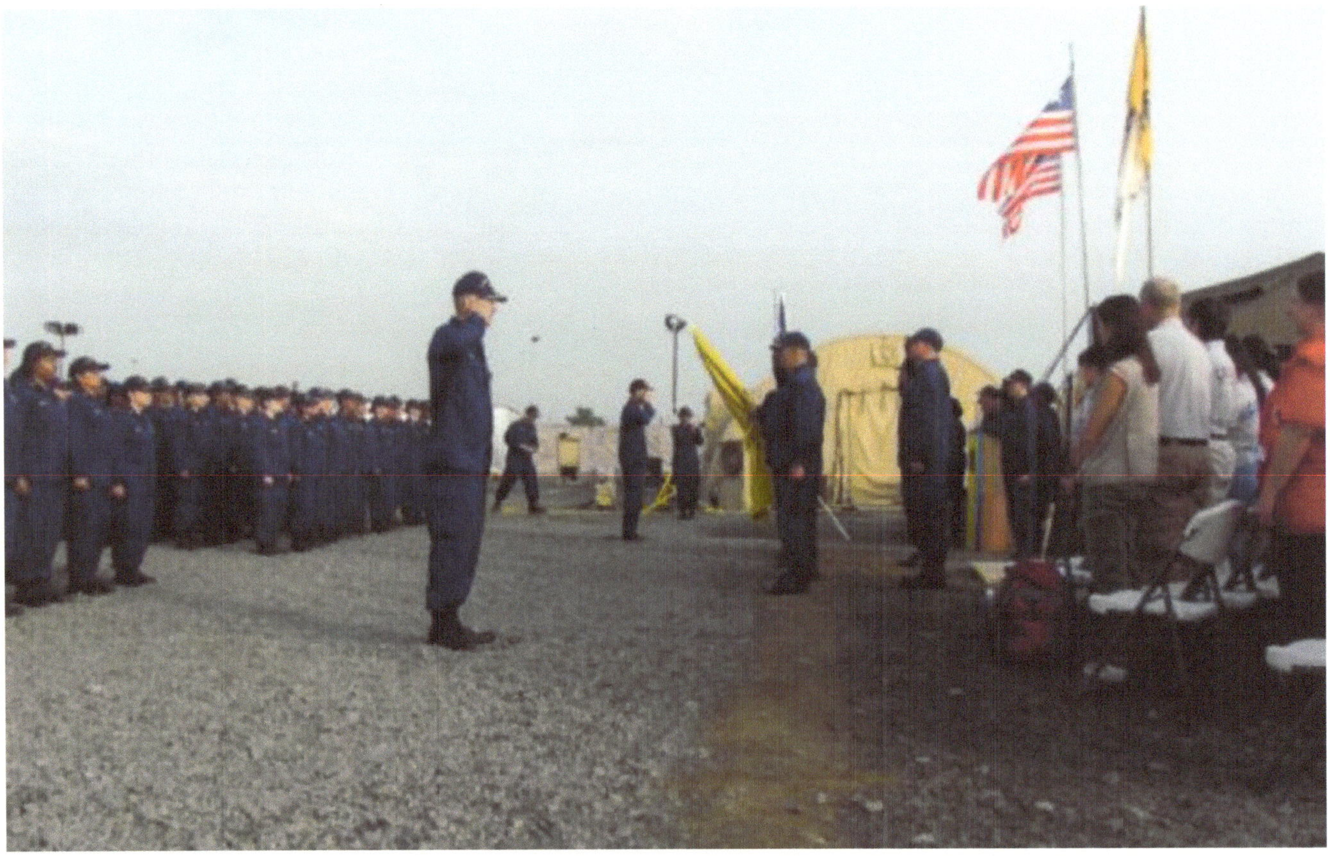

Preparation for the passing of the guidon. Right: The passing of the guidon is a time-honored tradition signifying the responsibility of command. In this photo, the outgoing MMU Team 3 Officer-in-Charge (OIC) passes the unit guidon to the incoming MMU Team 4 OIC, thus signifying the incoming OIC's ability to handle the responsibility of commanding the MMU in Liberia.

CAPT Rendi Murphree

"I remember thinking that no country is prepared to handle an outbreak of this magnitude."

—Rendi Murphree, MS, PhD

In September 2014, at the peak of the Ebola virus outbreak, CAPT Rendi Murphree, MS, PHD, served as the Centers for Disease Control and Prevention (CDC) consultant to the Montserrado County Health Team in Monrovia, Liberia. Monrovia was the hotspot of the outbreak. CAPT Murphree recalls that everyone was overwhelmed with morbidity, mortality, and intense efforts to monitor more than four thousand exposed contacts. CAPT Murphree recounts, "I remember thinking that no country is prepared to handle an outbreak of this magnitude. I observed case investigation and burial teams and provided recommendations for improvement, visited dozens of community health clinics to identify potential locations for additional isolation wards, and did my best to improve surveillance activities to better inform decision makers."

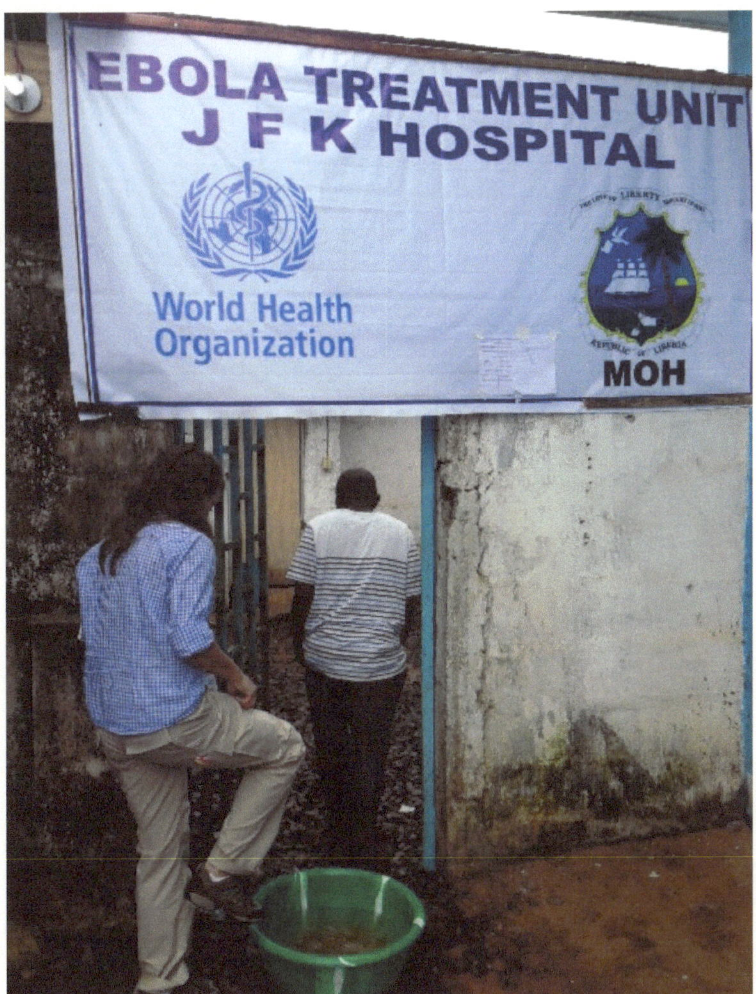

CAPT Murphree "disinfecting" the soles of her shoes before entering the ETU within the John F. Kennedy Hospital in Monrovia, Liberia.

CAPT Angela K. Shen

"I was impressed by the resilience of the Liberian community . . ."

—Angela K. Shen, ScD, MPH

CAPT Angela K. Shen led the routine immunization efforts at the United States Agency for International Development (USAID), as well as coordinated and led USAID's portfolio on routine immunization from 2012 to 2015. During the Ebola response, CAPT Shen was the USAID lead in the World Health Organization (WHO) Global Ebola Vaccine Deployment Team and a senior advisor to USAID on the US government's multi-billion dollar investment in the Global Alliance for Vaccines and Immunization, a multilateral global public-private partnership to improve access to and extend the benefits of life-saving vaccines to all, better known as Gavi, the Vaccine Alliance. CAPT Shen also supported the USAID mission's effort to rebuild and strengthen routine immunization systems in Liberia. She shares, "I was impressed by the resilience of the Liberian community in withstanding the challenges faced by the country after years of civil war that contributed to the country's weak health system."

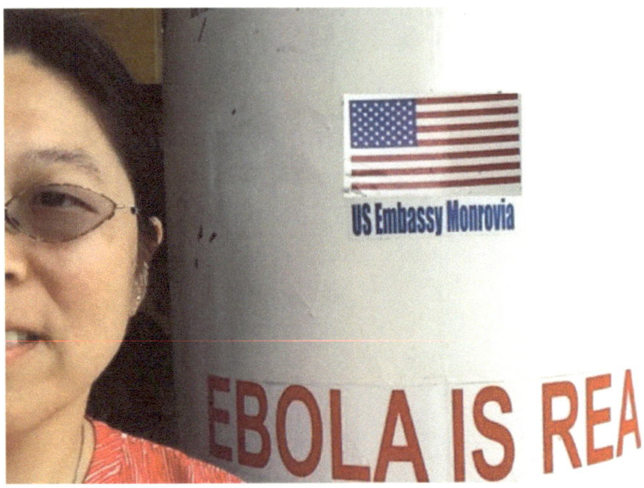

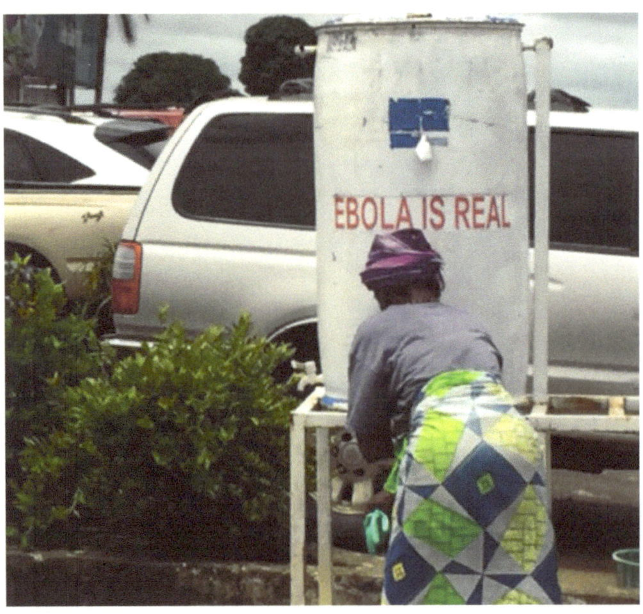

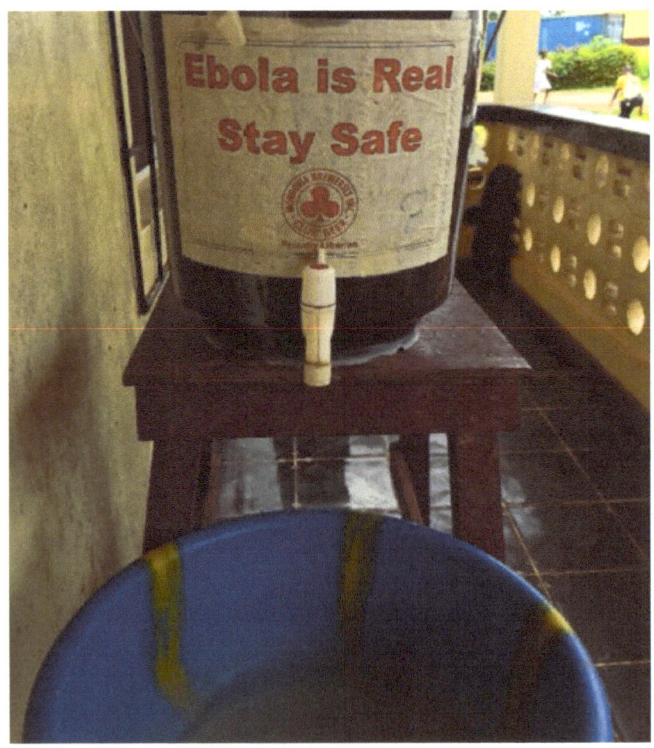

CAPT Shen captured the above photo of a makeshift handwashing station bearing the signage "Ebola is Real. Stay Safe." She also poses by the handwashing station *(above)*. *(left)* A local woman accesses the makeshift handwashing station.

"Faced with this outbreak, the world is looking to the United States, and it's a responsibility we embrace—to lead, to provide the capabilities only America has."

—*President Barack Obama, September 2014*

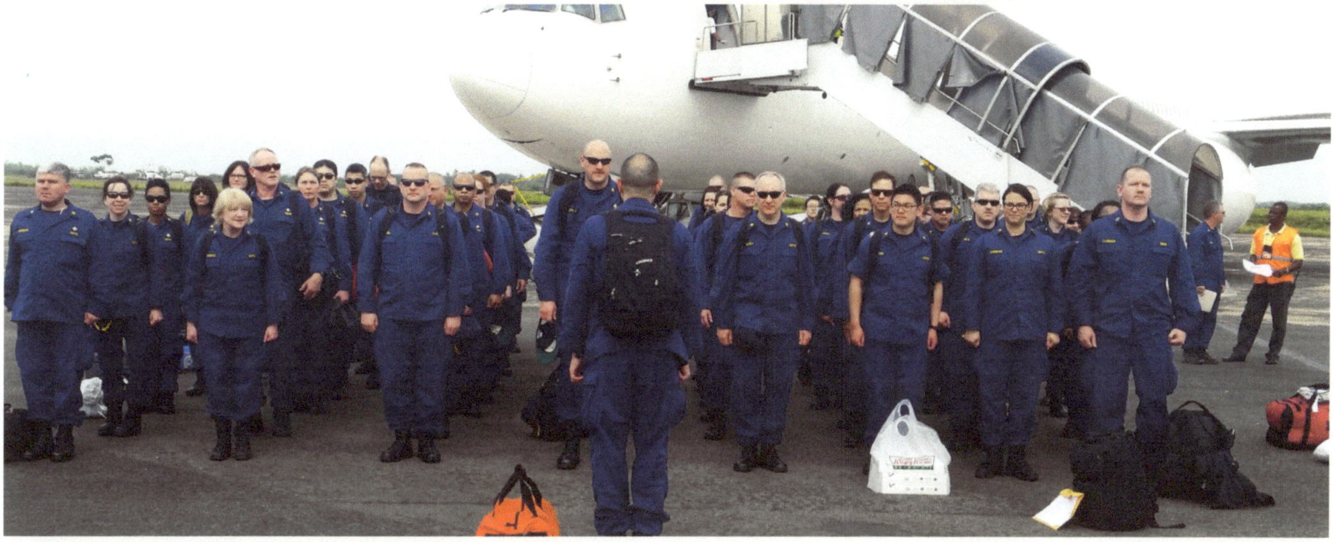

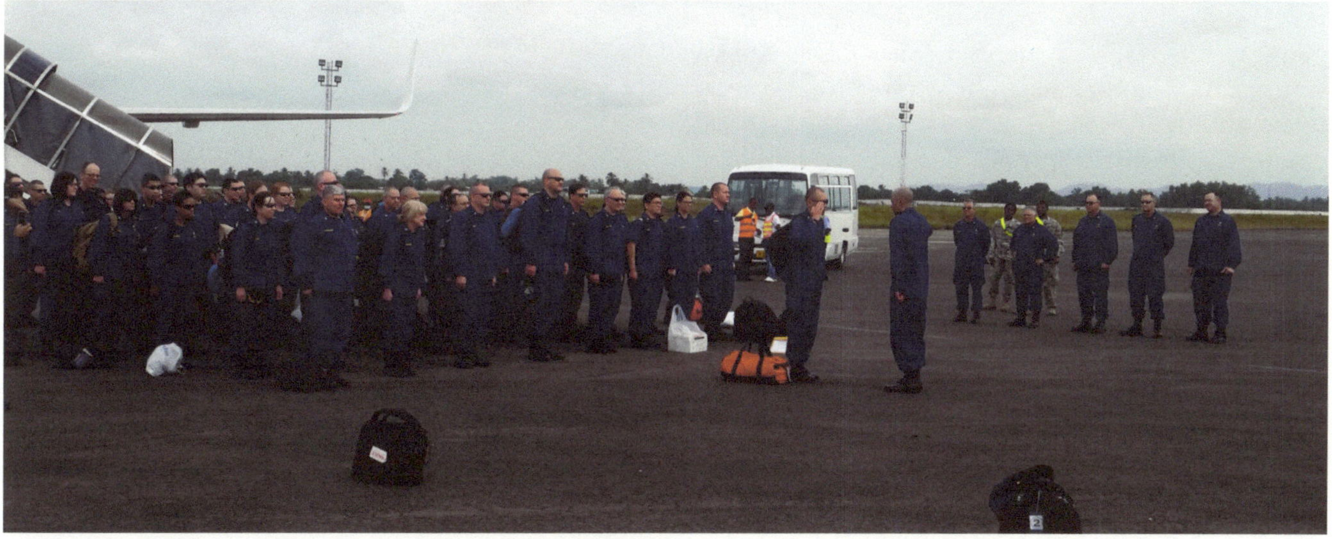

(above & below) Monrovia Medical Unit (MMU) Team 4 arrives in Margibi County, Liberia, to relieve MMU Team 3 from duty.

"About sixty-five Public Health Service officers are scheduled to arrive in Monrovia this coming week and could stay up to sixty days. They were handpicked for the mission and had the option of declining. But no one that was asked to go said no, according to a Health and Human Services spokeswoman."

—J. Achenbach & L.H. Sun.
"US Ebola Fighters Head to Africa, but Will the Military and Civilian Effort Be Enough?"

Originally published October 25, 2014, at https://www.washingtonpost.com/national/health-science/us-ebola-fighters-head-to-africa-but-will-the-military-and-civilian-effort-be-enough/2014/10/25/1ceba6a8-5b99-11e4-8264-deed989ae9a2_story.html

CDR Christye Brown

"As a non-clinician, it was a proud feeling to be able to screen passengers from the affected countries. . . . I also recall easing the minds of many of these individuals because it was an overwhelming time for some. . . ."

—Christye Brown, PhD, MPH, MBA

CDR Christye Brown supported the Ebola mission from December 2014 through February 2015 as a public health advisor at the Atlanta Airport Quarantine Station for enhanced entry screening efforts. This position augmented staff in the Centers for Disease Control and Prevention (CDC) Division of Global Migration and Quarantine (DGMQ). The experience was multifaceted and allowed for invaluable collaborations with the local county health department, airport leadership, and US Customs and Border Protection in order to streamline the process for travelers entering the nation from Guinea, Liberia, and Sierra Leone. CDR Brown states, "As a non-clinician, it was a proud feeling to be able to screen passengers from the affected countries. With the proper donning and doffing of personal protective equipment (PPE), I participated in direct patient care, taking temperatures and asking a set series of questions to each traveler. I also recall easing the minds of many of these individuals because it was an overwhelming time for some, considering they were pulled out of busy international customs lines and immediately given a facemask before being escorted over to the screening area." CDR Brown also remembers driving out to the tarmac to have a quick pulse check with public health service (PHS) leadership aboard the plane filled with fellow officers boarded for Liberia. Before CDR Brown's sixty-day deployment ended, she developed a standard operating procedure (SOP) for the PHA role at the quarantine station to ensure a smooth transition for newly-arriving staff serving in this capacity.

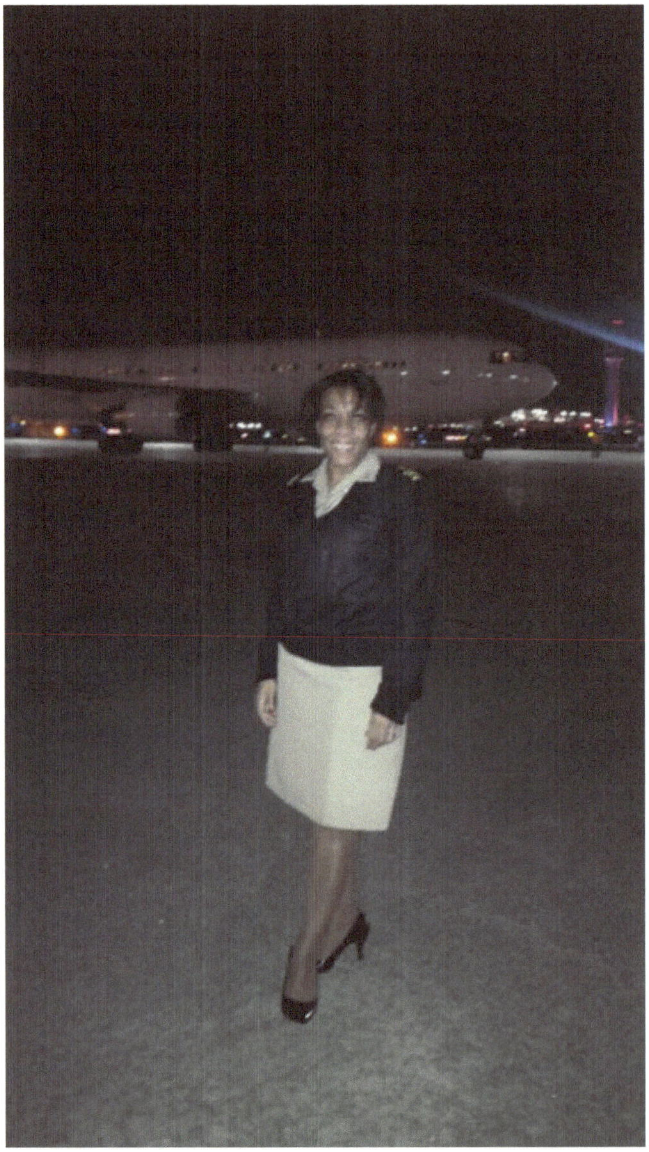

CDR Brown stands on the tarmac at the Hartsfield-Jackson Atlanta International Airport.

CDR Jacinta Smith

"Within hours of landing . . . I became a one-woman emergency operations center."

—Jacinta Smith, MS

CDR Jacinta Smith's first deployment to Liberia occurred in August 2014 at the early stages of the Centers for Disease Control and Prevention (CDC) field response to the Ebola outbreak. On the ground, she partnered with the Disaster Assistance Response Team (DART) to coordinate international logistics for personal protective equipment (PPE) and provide supplies to laboratories and airports in-country. In addition, CDR Smith served as an extension of the CDC Division of Emergency Operations, Logistics Branch, coordinating activities between Atlanta and in-country teams for support and services. Finally, CDR Smith assumed the activities of the CDC Liberia deputy team lead during a seven-day leadership gap. Her activities included forecasting the CDC in-country operational budget, auditing the Consolidated Overseas Accountability Support Toolbox reports, managing deployment rosters, and leading stakeholder engagement activities between the US Embassy in Liberia and CDC response teams.

CDR Smith recalls her first impression upon landing in Liberia during her first deployment: "As soon as I stepped off of the aircraft in Liberia to a bustling crowd of local media, government officials, and security, I remember thinking, 'We're not in Kansas anymore.' I intuitively knew that this outbreak was unparalleled to any response the CDC has supported in the past. Although the need was overwhelming, I was confident in our ability to successfully stop the Ebola epidemic once resources were mobilized to the region and systems were established in country."

CDR Smith also recalls that "within hours of landing on the ground, I became a one-woman emergency operations center! I served in a multitude of roles ranging from a medical logistician to provisional safety officer and finally deputy team lead during a leadership gap. As you can imagine, the early stages of an emergency response can be very fluid, so it was critical to adapt and learn quickly."

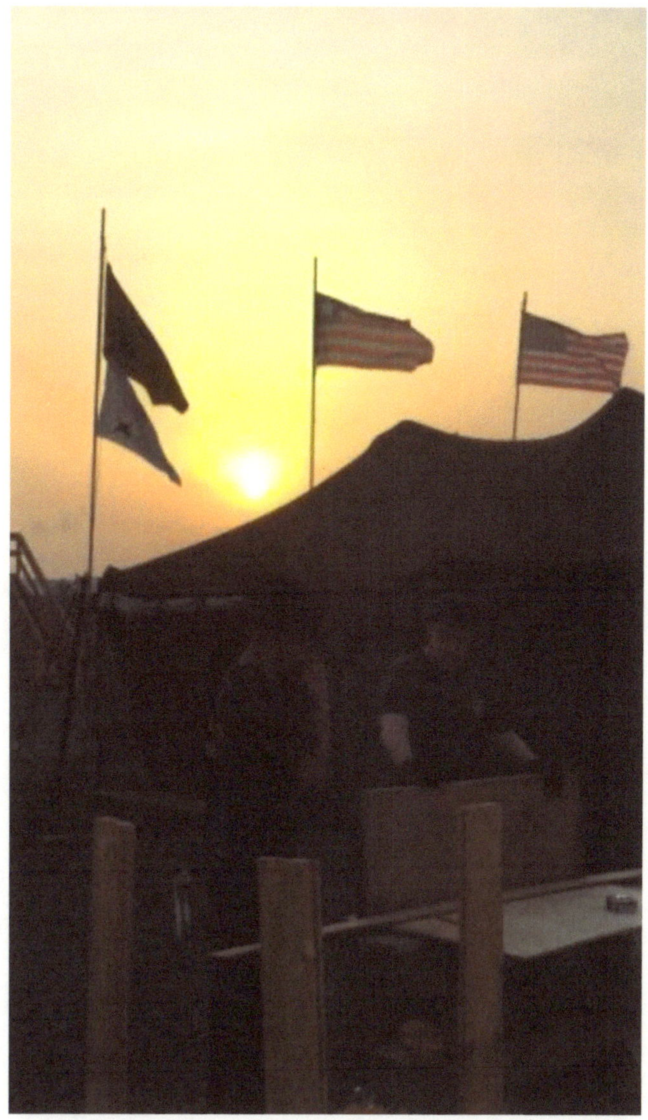

The sun rises over Camp Eason and the Liberian, American, USPHS Commissioned Corps, and Admiral flags. RADM Elizondo served as commanding officer for the Monrovia, Libera, Ebola response. Camp Eason serves as a beacon of hope to so many in the fight against Ebola virus disease (EBV) by providing high-level medical care for all healthcare workers who suspect they may have contracted EVD. Pictured: LCDR Gumapas *(left)* and LCDR Yang *(right)*.

CDR Smith deployed again the following year to serve as the CDC laboratory advisor in-country. During her second deployment, she coordinated personnel and resourced day-to-day operations of all Ebola testing in Liberia. This was the first Ebola outbreak in Liberia since the country was declared Ebola-free on May 9, 2015. The "Smell No Taste" Ebola outbreak was limited to eleven cases as a direct result of rapid Ebola virus detection, sequence data, and serology testing. Laboratory results were critical in defining the epi-link between cases and preventing Ebola transmission to Monrovia and neighboring counties. CDR Smith partnered with non-governmental organizations to develop the first Ebola rapid diagnostic test standard operating procedure and implementation plan for dead body management and safe burial teams in Monrovia. Development of Ebola rapid diagnostic test guidelines for clinical laboratories and dead body management teams across Liberia prepared the country to prevent, detect, and respond to emerging public health threats promptly. CDR Smith identified overall public health system improvements that could help prevent the spread of Ebola, which led to over sixty million dollars in cooperative agreements and resource allocation to strengthen and expand laboratory and health capacity in Liberia. In addition, CDR Smith developed a memorandum of understanding and data sharing agreements related to emergency public health response between the US government and the government of Liberia.

CDR Smith feels that participating in the Ebola response has been one of the most rewarding experiences in her public health career. She learned skills, shared experiences, and created friendships with members on her deployment teams that will last a lifetime.

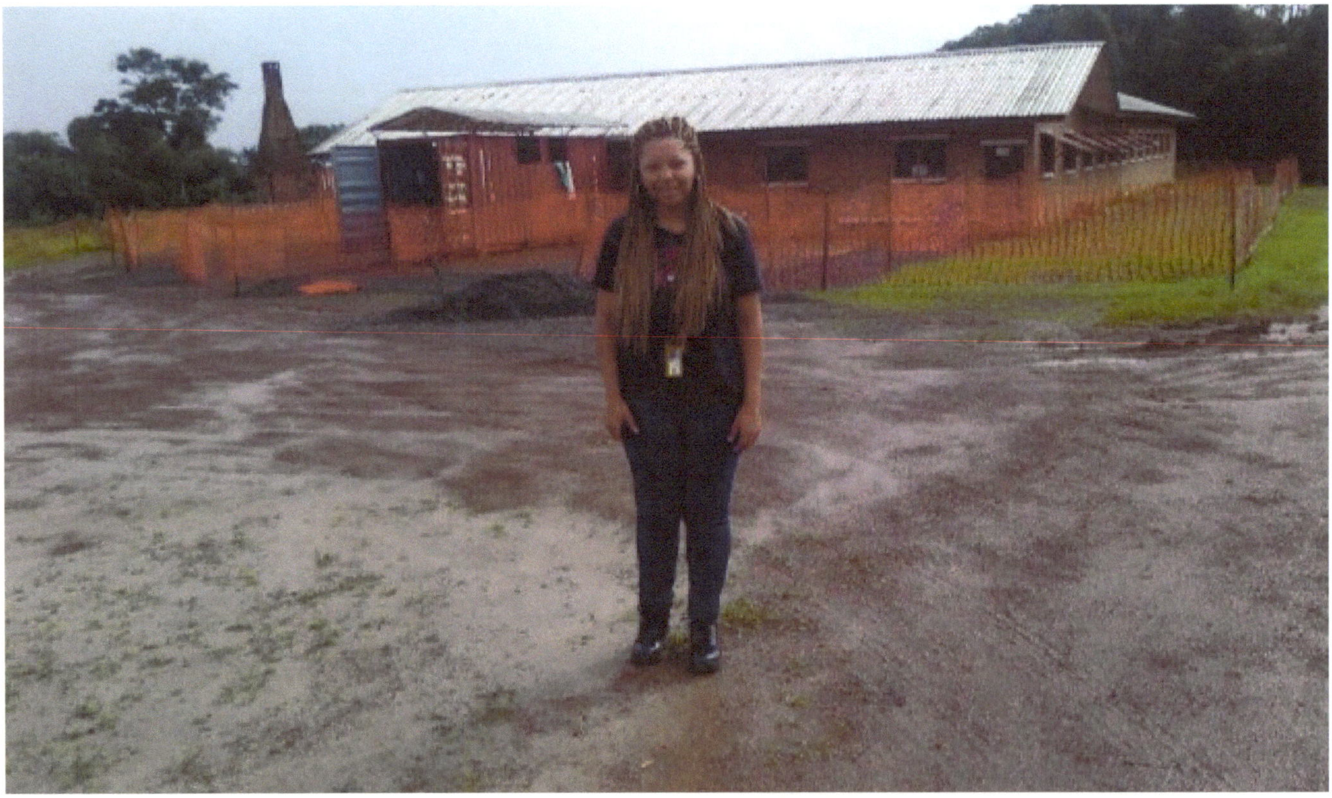

CDR Smith pictured in front on an Ebola Treatment Unit (ETU) at the Firestone Rubber Plantation in Margibi County, Liberia.

CDR Christopher Duncan

"All of these accomplishments occurred in a country with limited infrastructure where roughly 85 percent of the population lives below the international poverty line."

—Christopher Duncan, MLS

CDR Christopher Duncan was deployed to the John F. Kennedy (JFK) Memorial Medical Center, Monrovia, Liberia, from June 23 to July 31, 2015. He deployed via the Readiness and Deployment Operations Group in support of the Partnership for Research on Ebola Virus in Liberia III natural history study. The purpose of this ongoing study is to better understand the long-term health consequences of Ebola Virus Disease (EVD), viral persistence, long-term immunity, and whether previously-infected individuals can transmit infection to close contacts and sexual partners. The study—sponsored by the Ministry of Health of Liberia and the National Institute of Allergy and Infectious Diseases—was taking place at various sites in Liberia. CDR Duncan successfully trained five Liberian and three US laboratory staff, resulting in a cohesive and highly productive Partnership for Research on Ebola Virus in Liberia III laboratory operation during the initial stages of this important Liberia-US study. CDR Duncan recalls, "During my time in Liberia, over three hundred study participants were consented with approximately 1,800 blood sample tubes collected. In addition, I coordinated the installation and implementation of three new -80°C freezers at the JFK Laboratory. All of these accomplishments occurred in a country with limited infrastructure where roughly 85 percent of the population lives below the international poverty line." CDR Duncan felt that the most meaningful aspect of this work was an appreciative awareness of the many US government agencies and non-governmental organizations who work continuously to improve the health and well-being of the people of Liberia.

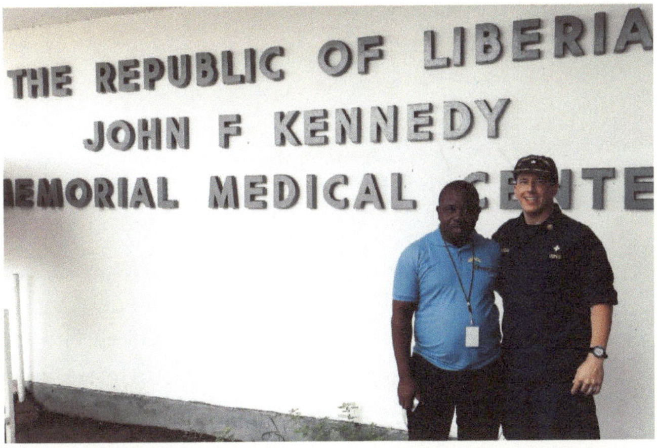

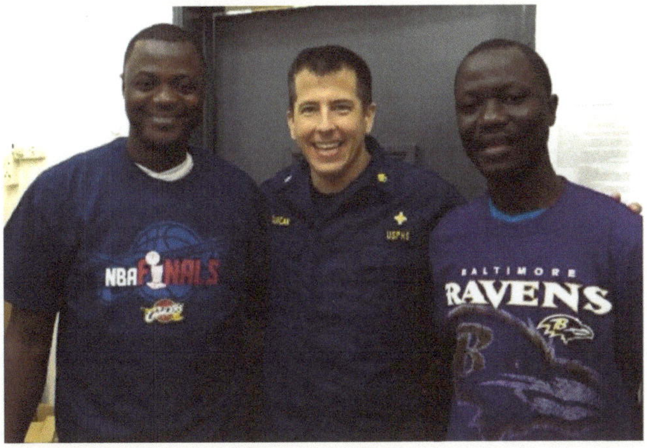

(right) CDR Duncan stands outside the JFK Memorial airport in Liberia. *(left)* CDR Duncan is pictured in the middle.

CDR Thomas Christl

"... working as the laboratorian for MMU Team 2 allowed me to have an impact on a much more personal and emotional level, making a direct connection with individuals struggling to survive. . . ."

—Thomas Christl, MS

CDR Thomas Christl was deployed as a laboratorian for Monrovia Medical Unit (MMU) Team 2. CDR Christl recalls, "It had been over a decade since I had done any active laboratory work, and that work had been environmental/marine research, but I knew I wanted to be a part of this response effort." As the director of an office of approximately fifty people, CDR Christl was very grateful to have the support of both his supervisor and the staff in his office. "I was also very lucky to have a supportive spouse who encouraged me to deploy. While I know that the work I do in the office has a significant impact on the public health of our nation, working as the laboratorian for MMU Team 2 allowed me to have an impact on a much more personal and emotional level, making a direct connection with individuals struggling to survive right across the hallway from my lab."

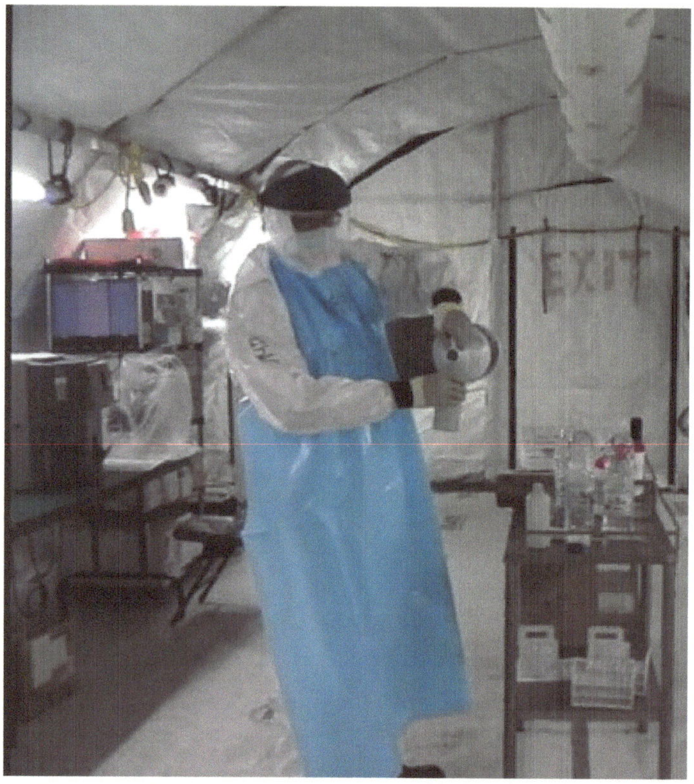

CDR Christl, in full personal protective equipment (PPE), runs the MMU Team 2 laboratory directly across from the patient treatment area. CDR Christl is pictured preparing the bleach solutions for the day.

CDR Christl describes those two months as an amazing and challenging time; something that will always be one of the defining time periods of his career and life. "As challenging as it was for me, I often recount that those two months were much harder on my wife. During that time, my wife had to contend not only with her high-stress job but also numerous problems with and around our house. In the matter of a week, we had an outside drain collapse, leading to basement flooding; frozen pipes that required her to smash holes in the drywall ceiling; our sump pump breaking during heavy rains; and a window in our master bedroom cracking all the way through, all with our dog in failing health (who passed two months after my return)." Despite the personal sacrifice, CDR Christl shares, "it was our duty and my pleasure to serve the people of Liberia, the international Ebola response effort, and the Commissioned Corps of the United States Public Health Service (USPHS) during that historic effort. I am grateful for that opportunity to serve, and even more grateful for the people and my support structure that made it possible for me to take part in such an important response and such an impactful experience."

CDR Debra King

"I was amazed how happy the people were despite having gone through a civil war, experiencing an Ebola crisis, and living in such poverty."

—Debra King, MLS (ASCP), MS

CDR Debra King was deployed to Liberia as the lead laboratorian on Monrovia Medical Unit (MMU) Team 3 from January to March 2015. Along with working in the Ebola Treatment Unit (ETU) laboratory, she was responsible for attending and participating in weekly meetings at the Emergency Operations Center in Monrovia for updates on the ongoing Ebola crisis. She coordinated with representatives from the Ministry of Health (MOH), Liberian Institute for Biomedical Research Laboratory, Eternal Love Winning Africa Laboratory, and other US and Liberian health agencies. CDR King directed all laboratory operations for sample collection and testing, and implemented laboratory equipment maintenance to ensure quality patient care. This proved to be especially challenging for a hot-zone laboratory where environmental conditions were far less than ideal. CDR King states, "Laboratory instruments create a great deal of heat; maintaining instruments in proper working order was very difficult, but I did it." One of her favorite memories was working out with her fellow officers each night to maintain physical fitness and general well-being while on a long deployment. She and her fellow officers would sometimes work out for several hours. CDR Debra King says, "I think we were all a little 'insane' doing Shaun T's Insanity Workout." After exercising, free time was spent trying to beat RADM Boris Lushniak in a game of Pass the Pig. In spite of these rambunctious activities, she also recalls, "The people of Liberia gave me the most rewarding experience. I was amazed how happy the people were despite having gone through a civil war, experiencing an Ebola crisis, and living in such poverty. I learned very quickly how fortunate I am and to not take possessions and life for granted."

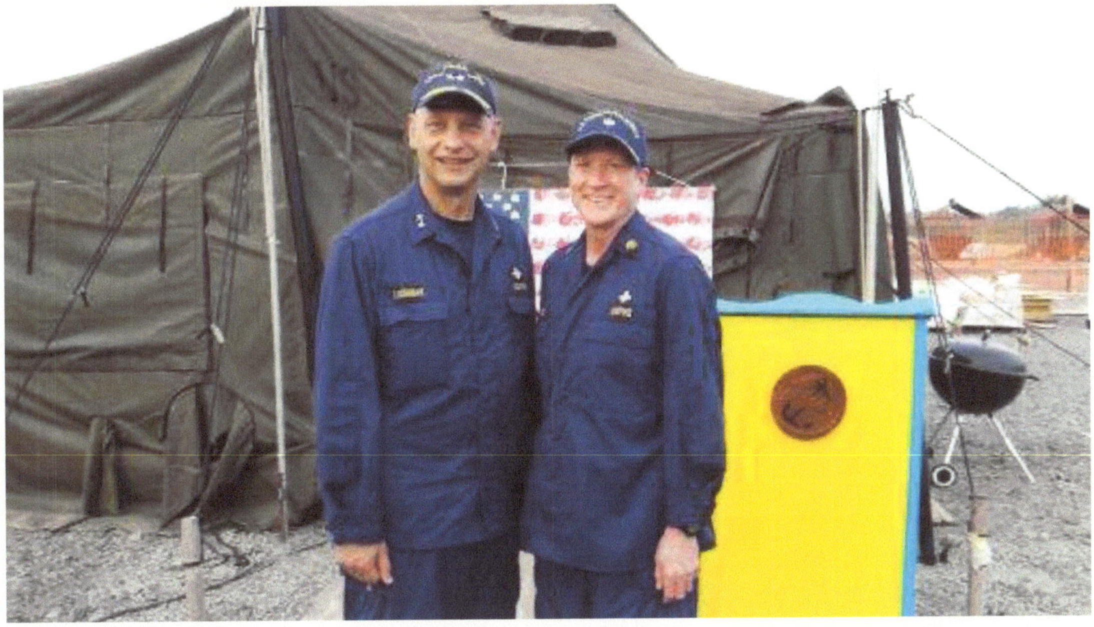

RADM Lushniak *(left)* and CDR King *(right)* pictured outside a tent in the Ebola Treatment Unit compound eagerly anticipating a night of Pass the Pig.

CDR Ericka Murray

"The day Liberia was declared Ebola-free, my heart was filled with pride and joy."

—Ericka Murray, MPH

CDR Ericka Murray deployed to Liberia in early December 2014 for sixty-five days. She shares, "The support I received from my agency (US Department of Homeland Security), my family, and friends as I prepared for my first United States Public Health Service (USPHS Commissioned Corps) deployment was amazing." CDR Murray served as a laboratory analyst at the Monrovia Medical Unit (MMU), which was located in an area of Liberia where the Ebola virus had tragically taken many lives. The MMU was the only facility in Liberia that was equipped with an on-site laboratory, allowing patients to receive exceptional, targeted care within two hours of sample collection. During this deployment, CDR Murray shares that she spent approximately seventy hours in full personal protective equipment (PPE) conducting rapid and point-of-care laboratory tests on patients. Her unique role allowed her to be among the first to see each patient's progress. "The day Liberia was declared Ebola-free, my heart was filled with pride and joy. It was my distinguished honor to serve with the USPHS Commissioned Corps, to be a part of history, and to make such a tremendous impact on the people of Liberia."

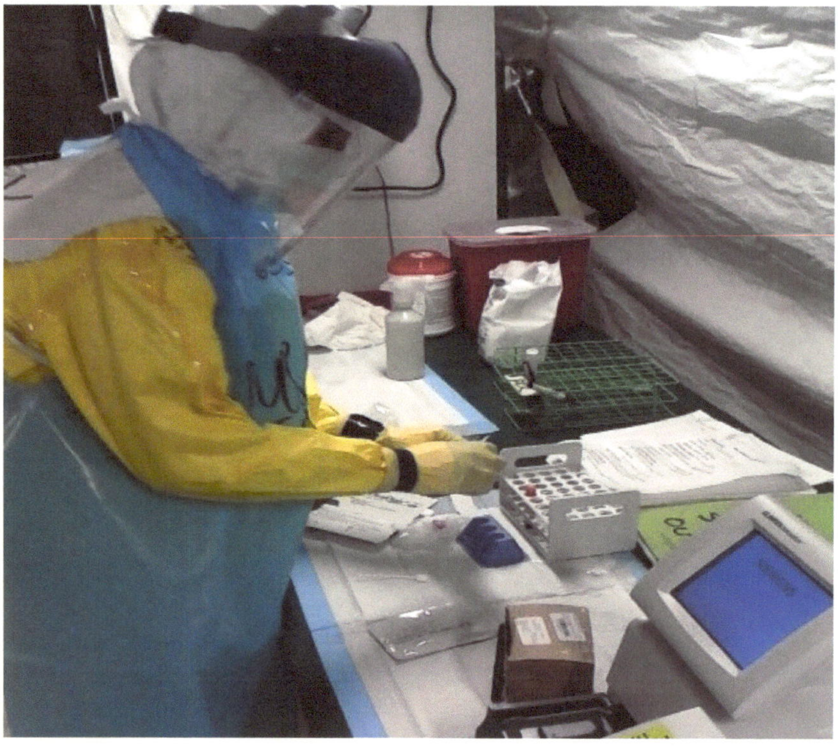

CDR Murray, laboratory analyst at the MMU, in full PPE conducting rapid and point-of-care laboratory tests on patient samples.

LCDR Jennifer Cockrill

"This interaction with my fellow officers, and facilitating their entry back to the United States, was the highlight of my deployment."

—Jennifer Cockrill MS, MPH, REHS

LCDR Jennifer Cockrill was deployed to Liberia as the Centers for Disease Control and Prevention (CDC) team lead for border health. As a border health specialist, or quarantine officer, her mission was to ensure that no cases of Ebola entered or left Liberia. She focused on the international airport and land borders that Liberia shared with neighboring countries. She recalls,

"As luck would have it, the end of my deployment coincided with the return date for Monrovia Medical Unit (MMU) Team 4, so I was privileged to brief MMU Team 4 ahead of their departure on the CDC's entry screening process and subsequently conduct their entry screening in-flight as we returned to the United States together. This interaction with my fellow officers, and facilitating their entry back to the United States, was the highlight of my deployment."

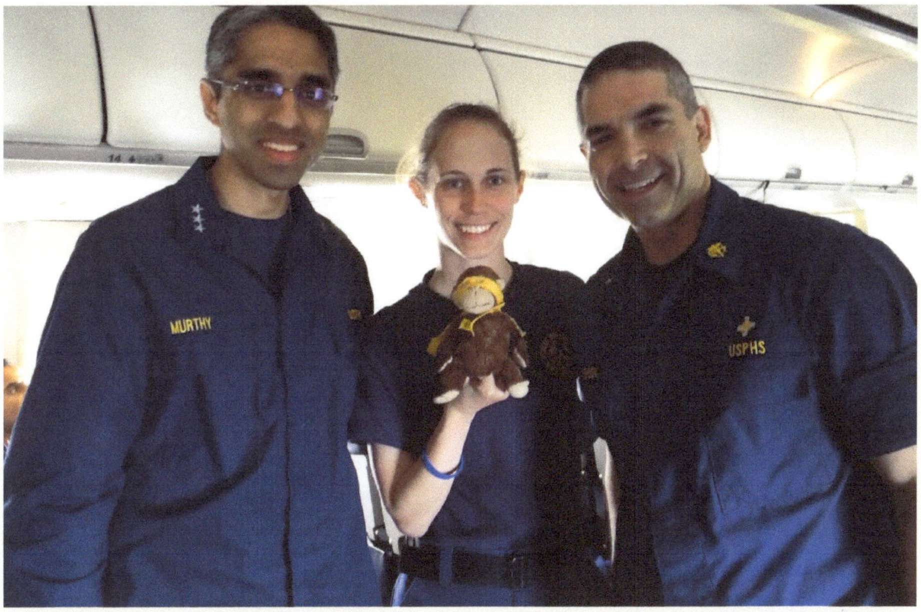

LCDR Cockrill stands between VADM Murthy and RADM Giberson holding the Quarantine Branch mascot (a small stuffed monkey) on the charter flight home to the US.

LCDR Elizabeth Garza

"[Our admirals] were extremely grateful to have 'one of their own' waiting on them after their deployment to the Monrovia Medical Unit (MMU)."

—Elizabeth Garza, MPH, CPH

Part of the first wave deployed with the Centers for Disease Control and Prevention (CDC) Ebola virus enhanced screening operations, LCDR Garza served at the CDC Quarantine Station at Washington Dulles Airport. While serving in this capacity, the Officer-in-Charge (OIC) asked LCDR Garza to accept the increased responsibility of day shift operations lead. She assisted with all parts of the response and accompanied the OIC when he met with airport partners. LCDR Garza was valued for her knowledge of the overall Ebola response, including the CDC's current role, the CDC's integration with Customs and Border Protection, and the greater role of the USPHS Commissioned Corps. She was often asked to assist with VIP tours ranging from Ron Klain, the Ebola response coordinator for the White House, to Congressional delegations. LCDR Garza recalls fondly, "Being deployed to the Washington Dulles Airport CDC Quarantine Station gave me a great sense of pride in not only being able to welcome home some of our very own officers deployed to West Africa but understanding more about our current role in quarantine and how that's evolved since our origins in the late nineteenth century where we had a Public Health Service (PHS) cutter ship to transport quarantine inspectors to board ships flying the yellow quarantine flag."

LCDR Garza's most rewarding experience was being able to escort several PHS flag officers returning from Ebola deployments. This included coming in during off hours and often meeting them planeside, or pulling them out of the sea of customs travelers to bring them to the front of the line and walk them through the Ebola screening process.

LCDR Garza shares, "I was able to meet RADM Anne Schuchat, MD planeside and drive her to where she was staying in Washington, DC, which was an honor, as she shared some insights on her experience and the situation on the ground. I was also able to personally escort RADM Sylvia Trent-Adams, RADM Scott Giberson, and RADM Boris Lushniak through the screening process and ensure they were home to their loved ones as quickly as possible. They all were extremely grateful to have 'one of their own' waiting on them after their deployment to the Monrovia Medical Unit (MMU). I was also able to meet an officer who had a family emergency and had to come home early and know how gratified he was during this tough time to have a friendly face at the end of his journey home to meet him and walk him through the screening."

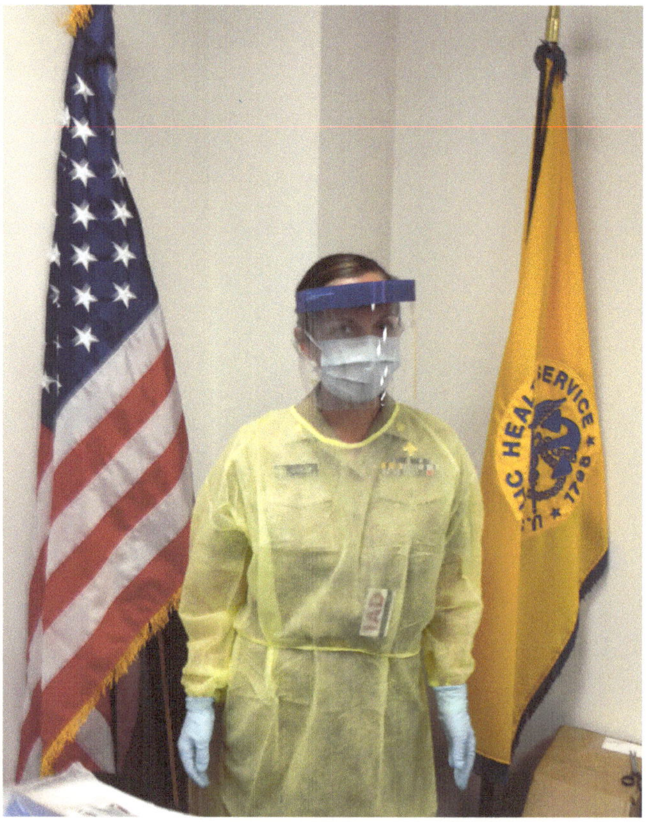

LCDR Garza working at the CDC Quarantine Station at Washington Dulles Airport.

LCDR David Hunter

"The lessons learned from these activities assisted the three other quarantine stations to fully establish the screening program for all inbound travelers from affected areas in West Africa."

—David Hunter MPH, MSW

During the Ebola outbreak, LCDR David Hunter supported the Centers for Disease Control and Prevention (CDC) response in three separate roles over the course of four months in the fall of 2014. He first deployed to Nigeria to assist with the implementation of traveler entry and exit screening from airports, seaports, and land border crossings. The CDC's Global Migration task force sent LCDR Hunter to assess and assist with standing passenger screening efforts at the Port Harcourt and Abuja international airports, as well as at three major seaport locations. LCDR Hunter collaborated with stakeholders, such as port officials, state health department staff, airlines, and clinical staff. He says, "These collaborations allowed for the development of site-specific protocols, the training of staff on screening procedures, and the use of infrared thermometers, as well as the initiation of screening operations."

Four days after returning from Nigeria, LCDR Hunter redeployed to the John F. Kennedy (JFK) Quarantine Station in New York City to oversee the evaluation components during the startup of entry screening for travelers arriving from affected countries. He also assisted with streamlining operations. LCDR Hunter recounts that "the lessons learned from these activities assisted the three other quarantine stations to fully establish the screening program for all inbound travelers from affected areas in West Africa." Upon returning from New York City, LCDR Hunter joined the State Coordination Task Force in the CDC Emergency Operations Center to support response operations in a variety of areas, including training, communications, and mental health.

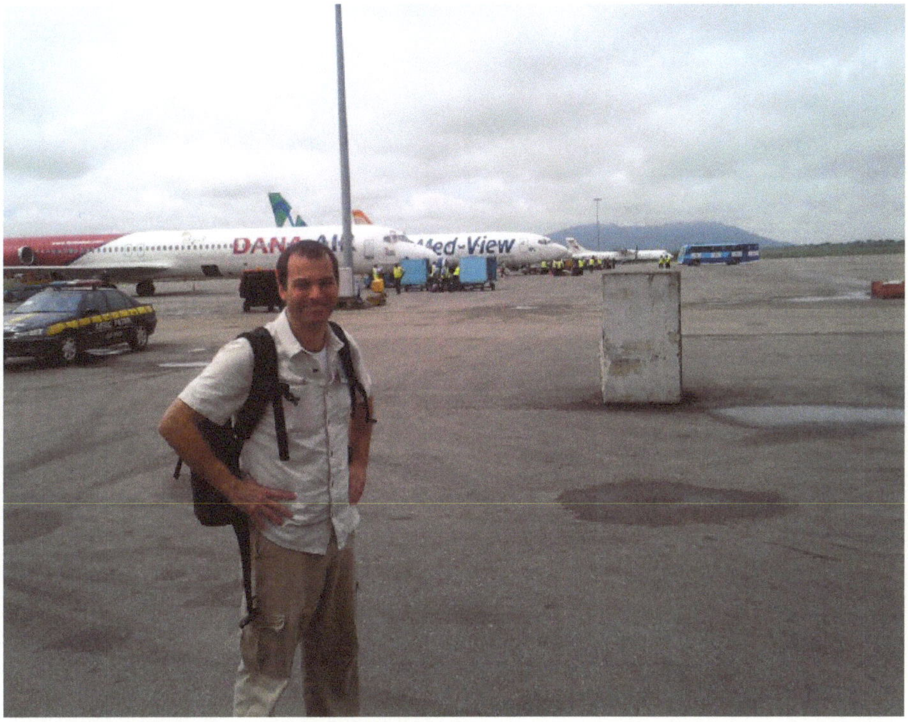

LCDR Hunter on the tarmac in Abuja, Nigeria.

LCDR Meredith Pyle

"Some days the drivers did not have gas, and they walked for eight hours to deliver the samples."

—Meredith Pyle, MS

LCDR Meredith Pyle deployed for two thirty-day missions to Bo, Sierra Leone, as part of a four-person team to perform diagnostic laboratory testing in a Biosafety Level 4 lab, which is the highest level of biosafety. LCDR Pyle recalls, "The greatest impact on me was being able to speak with the local people as they expressed their gratitude for my being there to do this work. I enjoyed working with the locals, who sometimes had to drive five hours on a motorcycle to deliver samples every day. Some days the drivers did not have gas, and they walked for eight hours to deliver the samples."

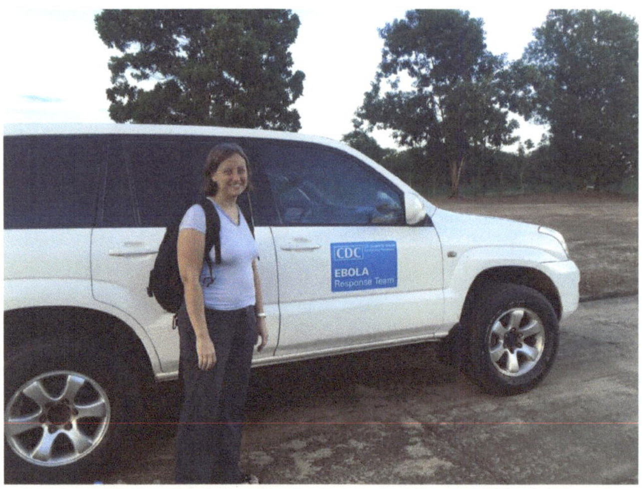

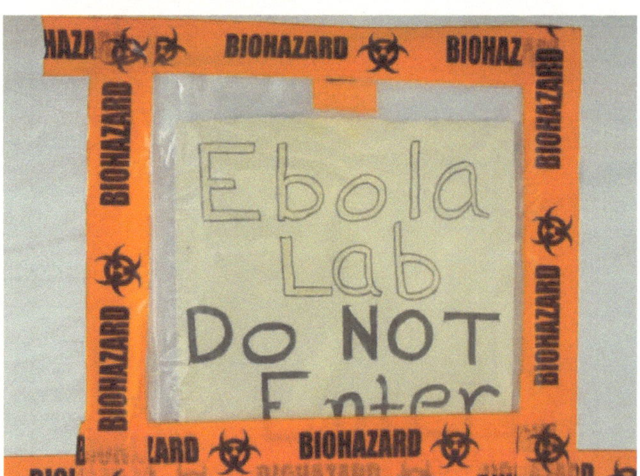

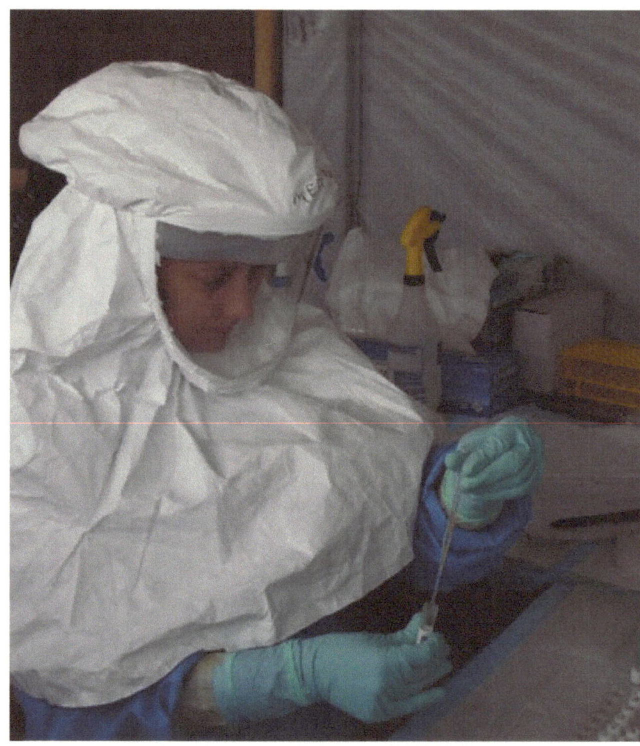

(top left) LCDR Pyle prepares to travel in a Centers for Disease Control and Prevention (CDC)–marked Ebola response vehicle. *(left)* Signage on the laboratory where LCDR Pyle worked provides a strict warning to passersby: Do Not Enter. *(above)* LCDR Pyle conducts testing in a Biosafety Level 4 field laboratory.

LCDR Osamede Onaghise

"It was the type of work that really put everything (even beyond the mission there) into perspective. It made me a better officer, husband, and dad when I came back home. . . ."

—Osamede C. Onaghise, MLS, BB (ASCP), MPA

LCDR O. Chris Onaghise deployed with Monrovia Medical Unit (MMU) Team 3 to Camp Eason, Liberia, as one of four lab officers from January 20 to March 25, 2015. The mission of the MMU teams was to care for healthcare workers that had symptoms of a possible Ebola infection. He explains that "the deployment seemed straightforward in theory—train for a week in Anniston, fly there, kick Ebola where it hurts, fly back. But the reality of getting there, the work, and the reintegration back to our lives at home was nothing remotely analogous to 'straightforward.'" The team surmounted some rather unique challenges before even touching Liberian soil and, once there, soon had to deal with the loss of a patient who had fought Ebola with all he had. They later shed tears of joy and relief as they discharged his recovering sister who had also been stricken with the disease and had endured the unimaginable fate of losing the sibling she once shared a tent with at the MMU—her battle buddy. The team treated and discharged a few other patients after ruling out Ebola. The role of lab officers was critical in all of this, as they provided a modest menu of tests to the clinicians and made multiple runs per patient to town to deliver blood samples for PCR testing at offsite support labs. Lab officers also wore a second hat as members of the Safety/Preventive Medicine team. LCDR Onaghise interfaced with a nearby US Army logistics team to acquire and maintain an inventory of blood products at the MMU. He also served on the morgue team and unfortunately had work to do there, too. LCDR Onaghise recalls, "It was the type of work that really put everything (even beyond the mission there) into perspective. It made me a better officer, husband, and dad when I came back home on March 25, 2015."

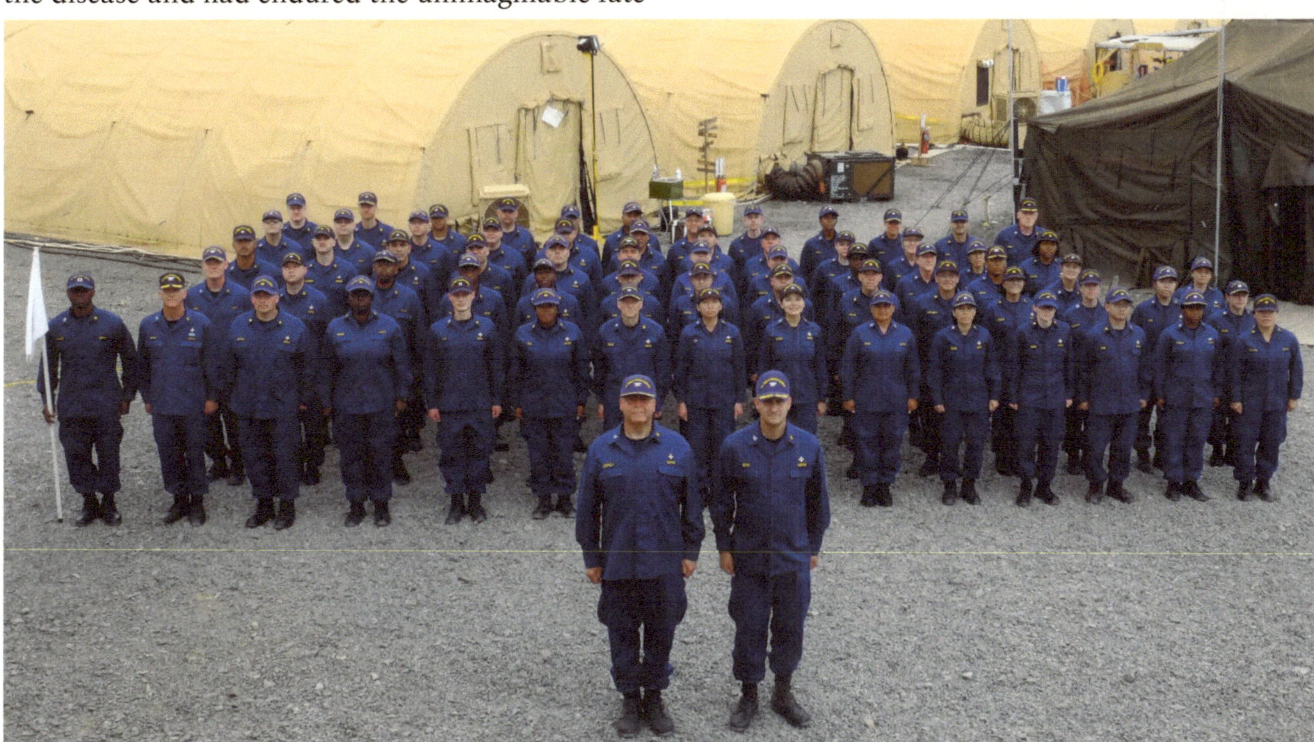

Monrovia Medical Unit (MMU) Team 3 stands at attention in formation outside Camp Eason, Liberia. LCDR Onaghise *(front left)*, holding the white flag.

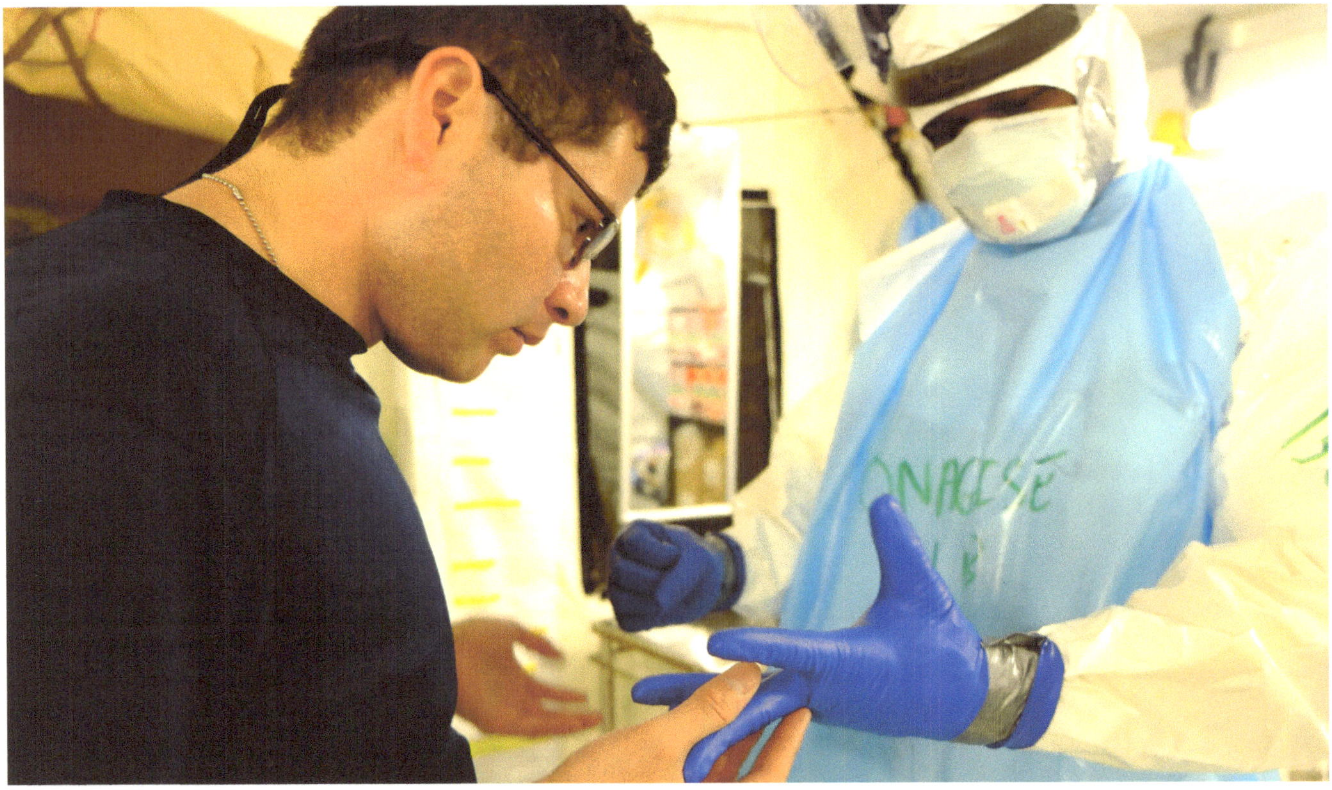

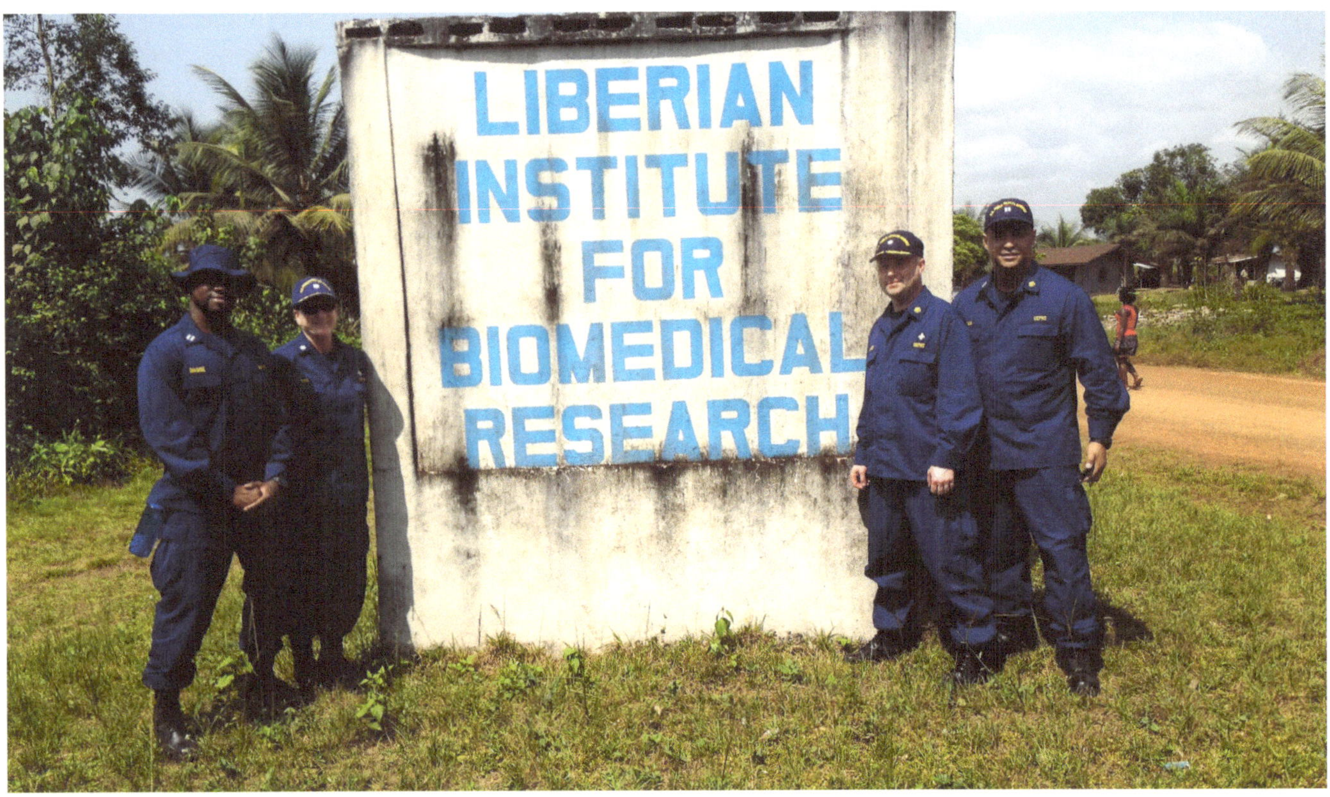

(top) LCDR Onaghise carefully examines his gloved hands for integrity as part of the safety protocols for the laboratory at the MMU. *(bottom)* LCDR Onaghise *(front left)* and fellow team members pose outside the concrete sign for the Liberian Institute for Biomedical Research.

LT Roberto Garza

"Given that the Ebola virus continues to be transmitted via breast milk, we were very worried that the mother, who was too poor to afford baby formula, would be forced to breastfeed, and potentially infect her child."

—Roberto Garza, MPH, MPA

LT Garza served as an epidemiologist and contact tracer in Guinea, West Africa from December 2014 through January 2015. He supported contact tracing efforts in the community of Matam in the capital of Conakry, including support for fellow contact tracers who worked in one of the other communities in Conakry. LT Garza worked side-by-side with local epidemiologists from the Matam Community Health Center to ensure that all contacts of cases had been checked and found to be asymptomatic and investigate any new potential cases of Ebola.

LT Garza recalls, "One of my best memories of this challenging deployment was when I was informed by my local counterpart that a woman who had survived Ebola was about to be released from the Ebola Treatment Unit (ETU) and would be rejoining her family soon. The woman had a three-month-old child who was waiting for her to return. Given that the Ebola virus continues to be transmitted via breast milk, we were very worried that the mother, who was too poor to afford baby formula, would be forced to breastfeed, and potentially infect her child. Our team immediately sought support from assistance agencies and other non-profits. We were able to share this need with an epidemiologist from Save the Children, a global nonprofit that improve the lives of children across the world. Our colleague successfully procured the necessary supplies, including formula, for this mother and her child."

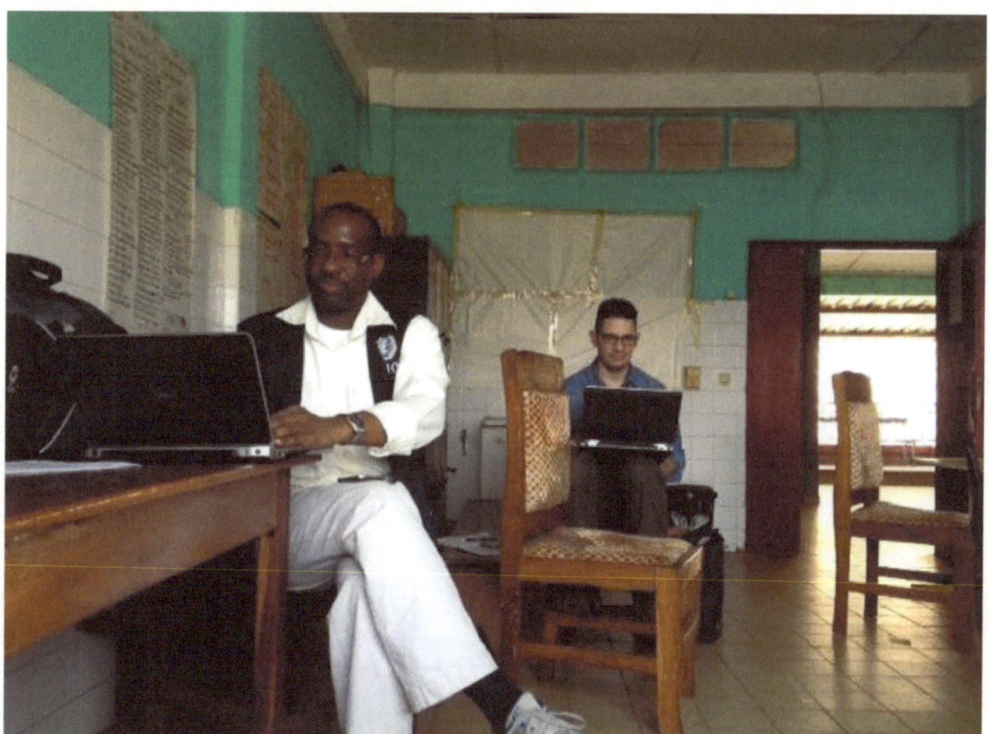

CDC's Varough Deyde *(left)* and LT Garza *(right)* work from the Matam Community Health Center in Conakry, Guinea.

LT Khadar Diria

"We not only protect the health and safety of America but also those underprivileged societies around the world."

—Khadar Diria, MS, MLS (ASCP), AMT

LT Khadar Diria answered the call from the Readiness and Deployment Operations Group (RedDOG) on June 3, 2015, to perform a temporary duty assignment in Liberia, where the National Institute of Allergy and Infectious Diseases, part of the National Institutes of Health (NIH), had initiated the Ebola natural history study in partnership with the Ministry of Health (MOH) of Liberia. The study was designed to better understand long-term health complications of Ebola survivors, to determine whether these conditions are the same or different from health problems faced by patients who have recovered from other life-threatening illnesses and whether survivors can transmit infection to household members. LT Diria served in this capacity from August 20, 2015, through October 10, 2015, at the John F. Kennedy (JFK) Memorial Hospital, the Duport Road Health Center, the C.H. Rennie Hospital, and the Redemption Hospital in Liberia. LT Diria, working as a clinical laboratory scientist, oversaw the operations of four clinical laboratories with a staff of twelve medical technologists. During this time, over 320 Ebola survivors and their close contacts enrolled in the study, and LT Diria supervised the collection of more than 1,900 blood specimens and over one hundred other bodily fluids. LT Khadar Diria trained nine Liberian medical technologists on proper interpretation of quality control results, troubleshooting laboratory analyzers, and laboratory data dissemination. LT Diria successfully completed the mission in spite of limited infrastructure, heavy rains, and persistent power outages. LT Diria recalls, "I was most impressed by the dedication and determination of the Health and Human Services personnel, and the USPHS Commissioned Corps officers in particular. We not only protect the health and safety of America but also those underprivileged societies around the world."

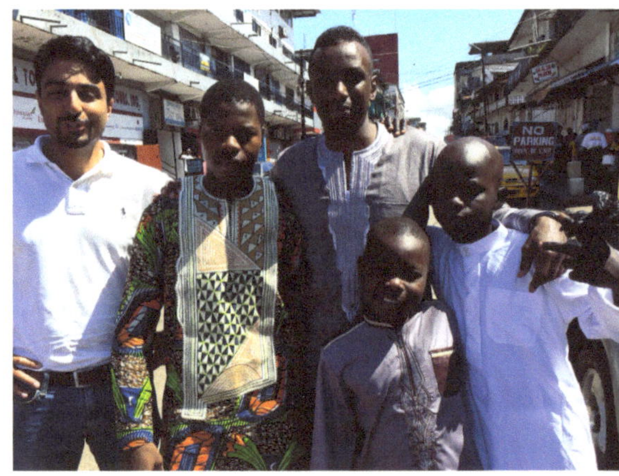

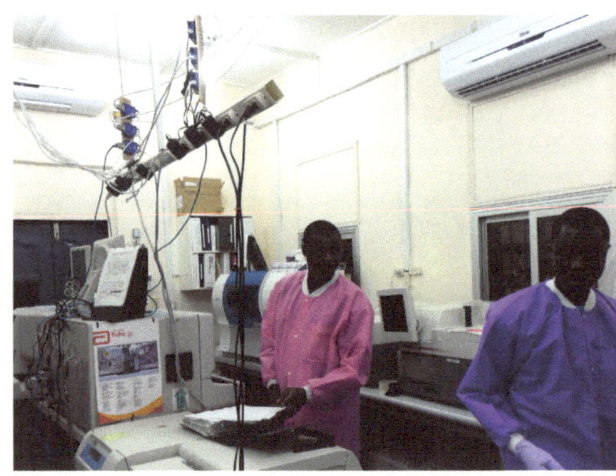

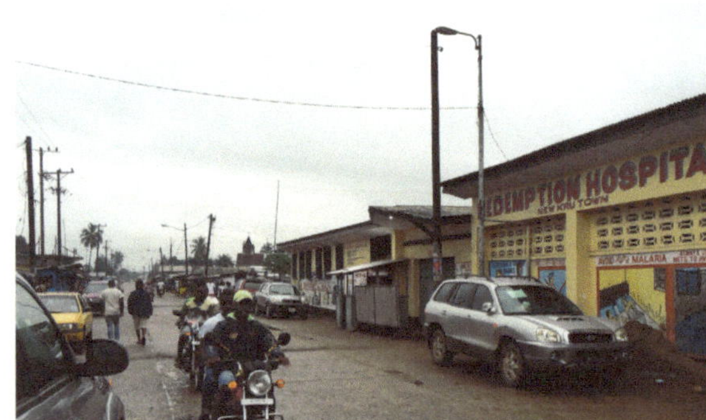

(top) LT Diria stands on a dusty street with several locals. *(middle)* Lab workers in the Redemption Hospital Laboratory. *(bottom)* A busy street outside of the Redemption Hospital.

LT William Brown

"While in the lab, handling samples at times was surreal."

—William Brown, MBA, MT (ASCP)

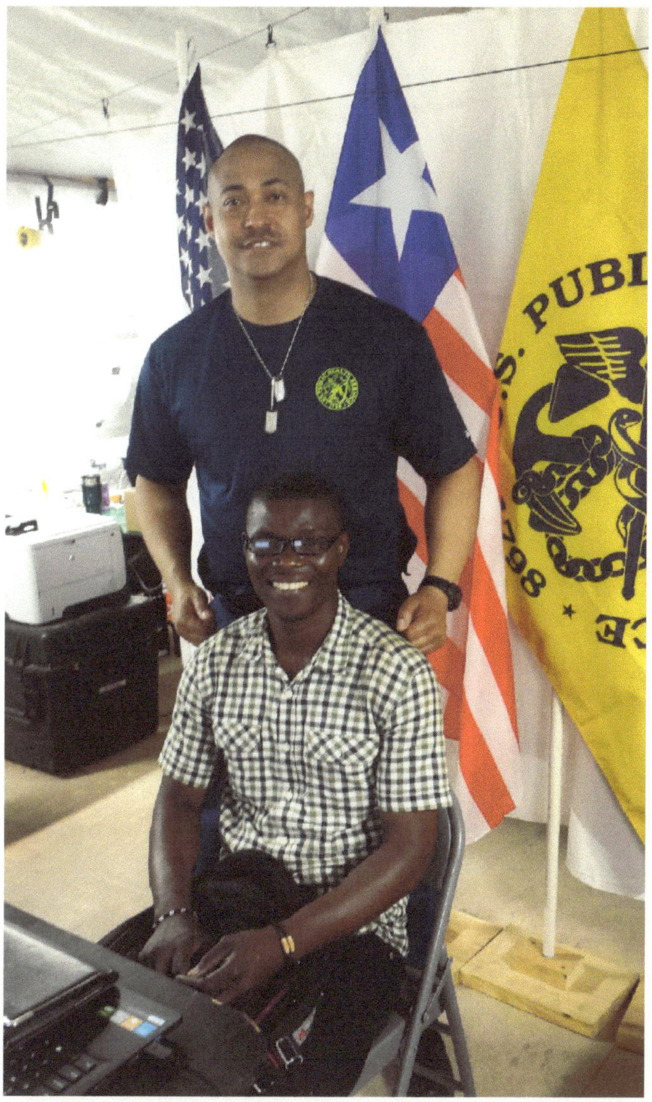

LT Brown (back) stands behind Alvin *(front, seated)*. Alvin is the first Ebola survivor of the MMU. As a survivor and a local, he was employed at the MMU as a valuable resource. LT Brown asked Alvin what he aspired to do now that he has survived his Ebola exposure. He said he dreamed of visiting the United States.

From January to March 2015, LT William Brown analyzed Ebola- and malaria-infected healthcare worker blood samples via complex laboratory procedures on several clinical analyzers for hematology, chemistry, and serology under austere conditions. He recalls, "Compared to a typical day in a United States lab, my team and I wore Biosafety Level 4 lab attire completely sealed in Ebola-level personal protective equipment (PPE)—Tychem suits, double-gloved, faces goggled and hooded, and rubber boots sealed with electric tape were worn within the tent lab. Blood samples that needed to be tested outside our lab were triple bagged with bleach solution infused between each bag layer before adding the item to a special sealed box, which was also bleach disinfected at the doffing exit. The samples were then transported to the Liberian Institute for Biomedical Research for Ebola and Malaria Analysis, as our camp could not house higher-level polymerase chain reaction analysis equipment, for it required stable ground and moderate temperature.

"The goal of our team was to treat and nurse Ebola patients back to health. Unfortunately, it was up to the patient's immune system and around-the-clock medical care to recover, as there was no cure or preemptive vaccinations at that time. Our lab was concealed and secluded in the hot zone next to the Ebola-infected patients. Compared to a United States–based lab housed in a building with HEPA filters, sealed doors, positive pressure ventilation, and temperature control, the Monrovia Medical Unit (MMU) used a tent system with no air flow, airtight room seals, ventilation, or temperature control, with a heat index exceeding one hundred degrees. The risk of heat exhaustion was so severe my team and I had to wear cooling vests under lab gear. While in the hot zone, my safety mask would fill with moisture, blocking the pores and limiting the amount of air intake. While in the lab, handling samples at times was surreal. I would make a mental note of the reality that existed between the immediate threat of Ebola contamination risk and the urgent continual need for protecting myself by practicing safety and universal precautions at a much higher level. Routine universal precaution alone was not enough! These extra measures and sacrifices were taken to protect the rest of the unit from exposure to the deadly Ebola virus. In a typical case, Ebola would cause morbidity within less than ten days. If an exposed patient survived the ten days, he or she had a possible chance of surviving. However, I did not want to experience trying to survive Ebola because chances of survival were slim. Staying calm while enclosed in the PPE under the heat in these austere conditions was a special challenge and learned skill. It became clear that as your heart rate goes up, more air is required, more moisture forms in the mask, and air intake is further decreased. Doffing takes a mandatory slow and detailed twenty-minute process to keep the camp safe from Ebola contamination. Focus, focus, focus! The lab was a team of four. We followed the guidelines set before us for how long each of us could spend in the lab to achieve the workload for the day. Ultimately, for maximum efficiency, we overlapped our entry/exit rotation one after the other by five minutes to brief the next shift until completion of our workload and laboratory practices. I made it a point to not have any emergencies relating to our lab team. Our lives and the lives of many others depended on it."

Upon returning to the states, LT Brown did not initially feel that he had changed much. However, after several days he realized he had unknowingly adjusted certain habits, beliefs, and practices. For example, he explains:

> "I will start with sleeping in my bunk. Oddly enough I grew accustomed to sleeping in a narrow bunk and raising to rotate. Currently I still raise and rotate as part of me still thinks I may fall off my bed if I do not rotate as opposed to rolling over. After seeing so many underprivileged lives, I learned to be more conservative, eat smaller portions, and make certain my plate does not exceed my appetite. I cannot find it within myself to waste food or water. 'Take only what you need' was a common statement made while at the MMU. I live firmly under that principle. As an officer I learned to depend on others. My battle buddy and the other officers realized the importance of supporting one another. We were all we had. That is a bond we will always share. I see the officers today at various Corps events, symposium, their agency in other states, and other deployments, and we always remember the experience we shared. We were a family and always will be. I learned the value of fraternity and sticking together under stressful conditions and holding each other accountable. My deployment to Liberia with my MMU brother and sisters has taught more valuable experiences and memories than I can count. These experiences and memories has added to my character. Bravo Zulu!"

LT Taran Pierce

"It was a whirlwind fifteen hours, and I never anticipated it would culminate in the most serious game of charades I had ever played. . . ."

—Taran Pierce, ScM

LT Taran Pierce deployed to the John F. Kennedy (JFK) International Airport in New York City from March to June 2015. She served as a public health advisor, conducting health screenings for passengers traveling from Ebola-affected countries. While on deployment, she implemented quality assurance processes for improving accuracy and completeness of screening reports, launched an enhanced reporting tool that increased the accuracy of daily reporting to Centers for Disease Control and Prevention (CDC) headquarters, and created dynamic inventory data system to track supply levels and request purchase orders. LT Pierce recalls,

"My very first day, I received training and then stayed after my assigned shift to assist with a passenger who required tertiary screening because it was reported that he spoke French. In fact, the passenger spoke Fulani, and the AT&T language line could not provide translation. We conducted the interview largely through miming and phoning a family member for translation via speaker phone. The physician I was paired with appreciated the effort I put in to ensure we had covered the full set of questions and could confidently release the passenger for remote monitoring. It was a whirlwind fifteen hours, and I never anticipated it would culminate in the most serious game of charades I had ever played—reinforcing that practicing public health requires commitment and creativity!"

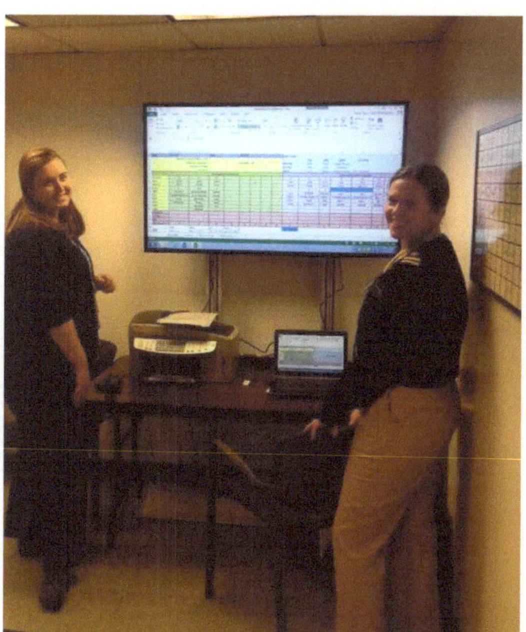

CDC employee responder Teneale Chapton and LT Pierce review the electronic flight board in Terminal 1 of the JFK airport.

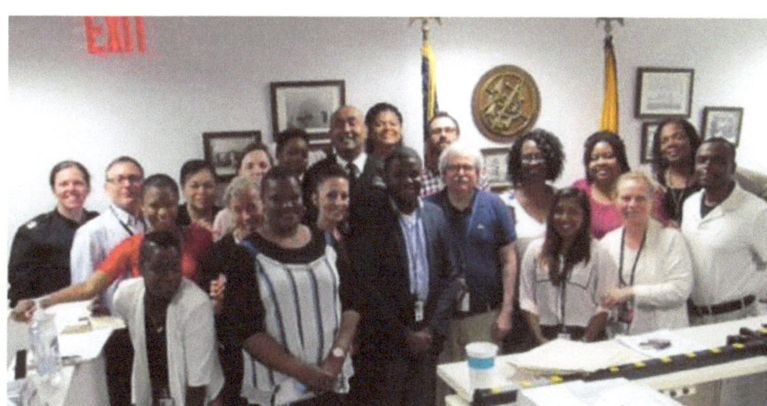

LT Pierce *(far left, back row)* stands with fellow Ebola responders at the JFK International Airport Quarantine station in June 2018.

The third pillar in the Global Health Security framework is the ability to respond timely and sufficiently to a biological threat such as Ebola. Response capacity is often highly dependent upon economic stability, access to critical supplies and medications, and the presence of subject matter experts to inform, guide and direct activities. Response actions of officers during the outbreak included the establishment and staffing of temporary medical treatment units, provision of technical expertise to strategic governmental and non-governmental posts to inform and support response coordination; and the training and empowerment of populations served to increase their internal capacity for future response. The following stories have been selected to demonstrate critical response activities from treatment of Ebola infected health care workers to the leadership support for incident command structures coordinating a joint response effort. This final section of stories is introduced by 2016 HSPAC Chair CDR Bobby Rasulnia who oversaw the successful conclusion of the response. In addition, it features a Force Leadership Highlight by RADM Epi Elizondo who directly oversaw the USPHS medical response to support health care workers for teams 3 and 4 at the Monrovia Medical Unit. The officer accounts of their work and the impact of participating in these response efforts are presented following military custom with the highest-ranking officers given the floor first in presentation. Some stories included in the section may have activities that span all three pillars of Global Health Security (prevent, detect, respond) but they have been placed here for the demonstrable evidence of response coordination and direct patient care.

A NOTE TO THE READER: *The Monrovia Medical Unit (MMU) features prominently in the stories located in this section. Some officers refer to it in their accounts as MMU and others as Camp Eason. The MMU was officially named Camp Eason on January 1st, 2015 during a naming ceremony lead by MMU Team 2 Officer-in-Charge, CAPT James Dickens. A hand-carved Liberian wooden sign designating the name of the facility was placed at the entrance. CAPT John Eason, Jr., in 1943, was the first African American to be commissioned by the United States Public Health Service (USPHS). Commissioned as an Environmental Health Officer, he worked as an assistant sanitarian for the Baltimore City Health Department. In 1945, CAPT Eason was selected to serve as liaison officer to the U.S. mission to Liberia. CAPT Eason was one of the first USPHS Officer's assigned to the Office of International Health where he supervised and supported health care missions to various countries all around the world. After 30 years of service, CAPT Eason retired in 1974. Through his USPHS career and into his retirement, CAPT Eason continued to demonstrate leadership, dedication, and commitment to the mission of the USPHS. Because of his officership, his ties to Liberia, and a few of the key characteristics for which he is remembered: leadership, dedication and commitment—the MMU Team 2 was honored to dedicate the MMU in the name of CAPT John C. Eason, Jr. The historic Camp Eason wood carving is now hanging in the renowned National Institutes of Health Clinical Center in a permanent display paying tribute to the USPHS Ebola Crisis Response.*

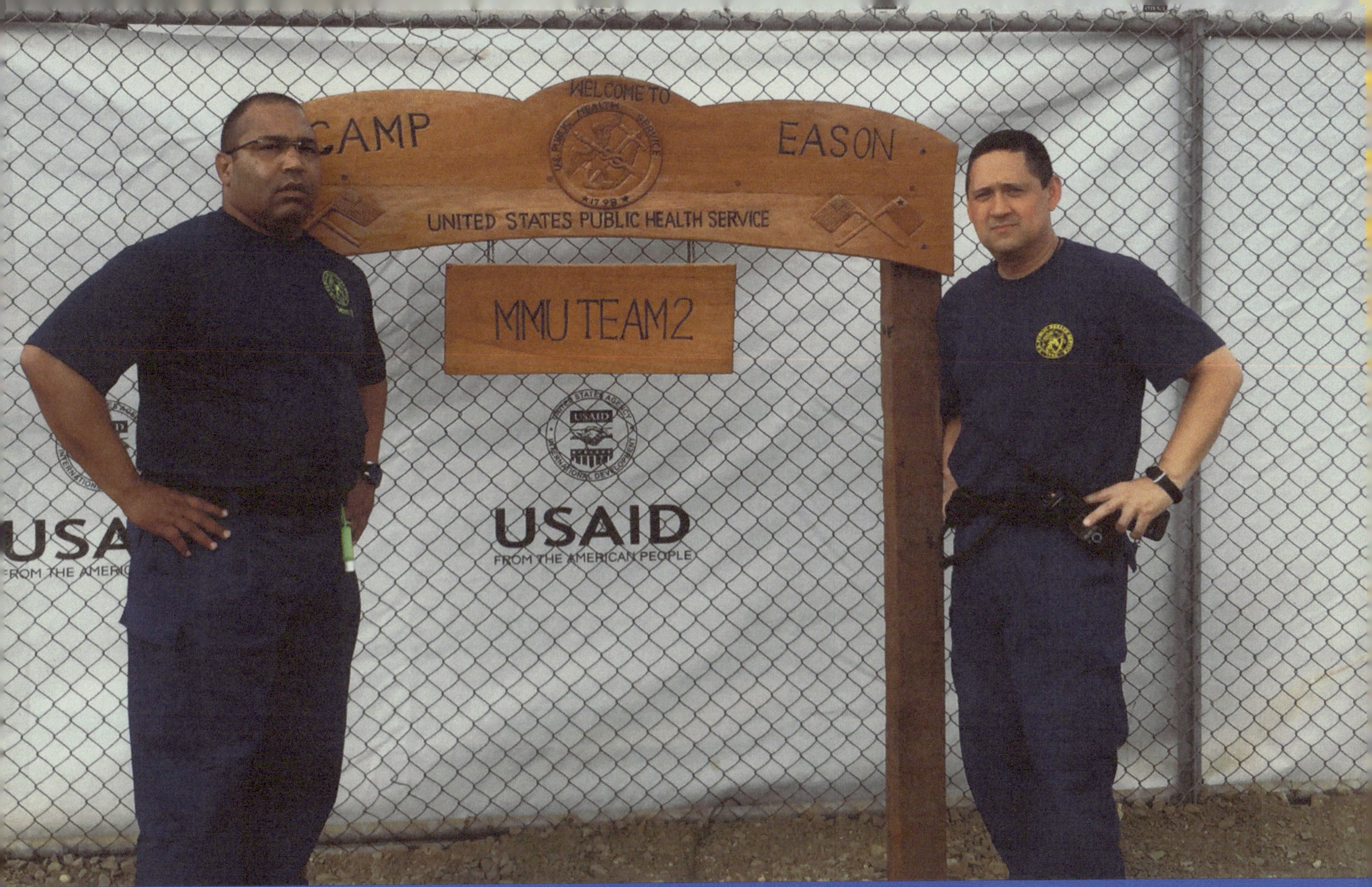

RESPOND

"Health services officers' response to the Ebola epidemic demonstrated dedication to the health and safety of others. While serving as a part of the Monrovia Medical Unit (MMU) team, these officers assumed several roles, including command, planning, patient care, preventive medicine, and behavioral health. This elite group of officers participated in the care of healthcare workers who were infected with the deadly virus while caring for Ebola patients."

Karen Forbes, MPA-S, PA-C
CDR, USPHS

(left) CAPT Dickens, Officer-in-Charge (OIC) and right: CAPT de la Cruz (Deputy OIC) of MMU Team 2 standing by the Camp Eason sign that was designed and erected by LT Pesce, LT Deckert, LT Holshue, and LT Sheedy.

HSPAC CHAIR: Perspective as the Mission Completes

CDR Bobby Rasulnia spent twelve months working on the 2014–2016 Centers for Disease Control and Prevention (CDC) Ebola response, serving in four distinct roles. "From my desk at CDC Headquarters in Atlanta, I served as the emergency coordinator for the Center for State, Tribal, Local, and Territorial Support (CSTLTS). In that role, I coordinated requests for staff to participate in the response, acted as the liaison between CSTLTS and Incident Management System (IMS) leadership for review of policy and communication documents related to states and localities, and coordinated Ebola data collection requests and Office of Management and Budget clearances in collaboration with the IMS Scientific Response section. My second role in the response was working with the IMS Deployment Risk Mitigation Unit. I implemented health and safety activities for CDC responders deploying to West Africa by providing guidance, liaising with them throughout their deployments, and working to address the stigma that they and their family members experienced after coming home from an Ebola-affected country.

> **"Experience can't be taught, it must be lived: DEPLOY!"**
>
> —Bobby Rasulnia *PhD, MPA, MPH, CHES*
> *CDR, USPHS*
> *Health Services Professional Advisory Committee (HSPAC) Chair, 2016*

"After ten months stateside, I deployed to Liberia as part of the Infection Prevention and Control (IPC) Team. I spent five weeks working in rural Liberia, where resources and communication were scarce. My primary role in Liberia was to assess how IPC protocols were being implemented in healthcare facilities; to train clinicians and public health workers on how to use infection control supplies, such as gowns and gloves; and to conduct clinic site visits. I also helped to evaluate the construction of two local Emergency Operation Centers. While in Liberia, I gathered Ebola Virus Disease (EVD) surveillance data, conducted surveillance training with public health professionals in-country and participated in an investigation into why livestock were dying in a community on the border with Guinea. I visited border health sites at Liberian border crossings with Guinea and Sierra Leone, which can each see over two thousand people crossing in a single day. Midway into my deployment, the World Health Organization (WHO) requested assistance from the CDC to support an integrated measles, deworming, and polio vaccination campaign. The Ebola outbreak had disrupted and strained the healthcare system in Liberia, which lead to outbreaks of measles, so I conducted site visits and monitored and mobilized the community to increase vaccination rates among children and prevent the spread of measles. After five weeks in the field, I returned to Monrovia to lead the Logistics Team. In this role, I interfaced with the United States Embassy in Liberia to ensure that deployed CDC staff had the logistics support they needed to travel safely and efficiently throughout the county. I was also accountable for the transportation of all CDC responders in and out of Liberia. Upon returning home, I realized that I wanted to pursue a new career path. The response had changed me for the better; it took me back to why I wanted to pursue a career in the public health in the first place. A year after I returned from Liberia, I became a permanent member of the Deployment Risk Mitigation Unit (now the Office of Risk Management and Operational Integrity), which was converted from a taskforce in the IMS to a permanent office in the Division of Emergency Operations. In this new role, I have continued the work that I started while working on the Ebola response to build capacity among CDC responders and improve the CDC's preparedness and response capabilities."

Bobby Rasulnia, PhD, MPA, MPH, CHES

CDR, USPHS
HSPAC Chair, 2016

During the response, then-CDR Rasulnia served the Center for State, Tribal, Local, and Territorial Support (CSTLTS) at the CDC in Atlanta, Georgia, as a health scientist. He led the Health and Human Services and CDC award-winning Office of Management and Budget Clearance Center, a three-year mechanism for collecting evaluation data from state, tribal, local, and territorial government staff and delegates for CDC programs. In 2015, he served on a short-term assignment to Kenya to operationalize and implement CDC-Kenya, an Africa Global Health Security Agenda program. Currently, CAPT Rasulnia serves the Division of Emergency Operations to the Office of Risk Management and Operational Integrity as the deputy director. He manages the day-to-day operations and programs of the office and provides strategic leadership and administration of a comprehensive risk-management program for emergency response operations and responders. CAPT Rasulnia has a PhD from the University of Alabama, concentrating in health behavior and policy. He also holds a master of public administration, a master of public health in community health, a bachelor of arts in psychology, and a bachelor of science in Biology, each from the University of Tennessee at Knoxville.

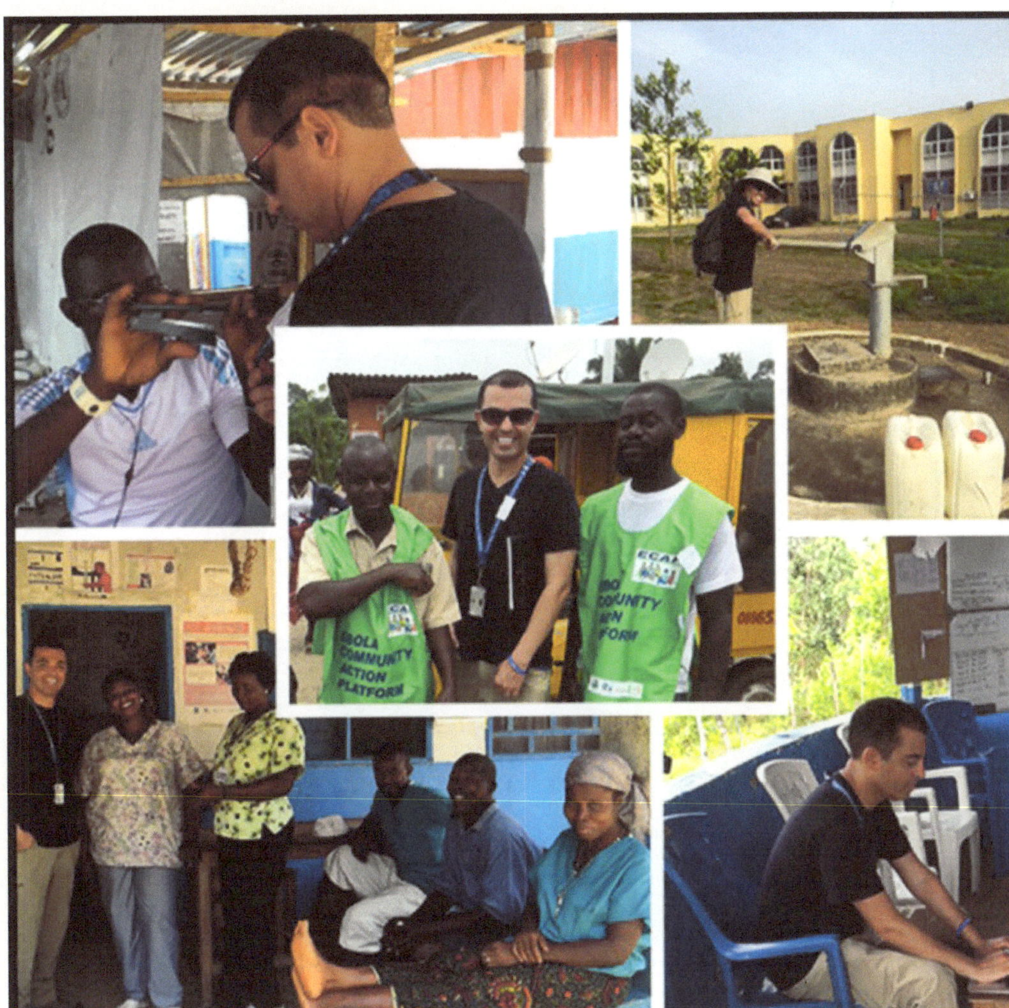

CDR Rasulnia is pictured in the black t-shirt in the photo collage above. CDR Rasulnia is seen working and interacting with the local public health community.

Force Leadership Highlight

RADM Epi Elizondo

"It was one of most exciting experiences in uniform, and I will forever appreciate being entrusted to serve as commander of the Ebola response along with other health services officers."

—Epi Elizondo, PhD, PA-C, DFAAPA

As the Liberia response commander for the Commissioned Corps Ebola Response, RADM Epi Elizondo had responsibility for oversight of the Monrovia Medical Unit (MMU) from February to April 2015. He worked directly with the US ambassador, the Liberian Ministry of Health (MOH), the Disaster Assistance Response Team (DART), the US Department of Defense (DOD), the National Institutes of Health (NIH), and the Centers for Disease Control and Prevention (CDC) to ensure open communication and consistent outreach for fluid response by clinicians when needed.

"Upon my arrival to Liberia I took over from RADM Boris Lushniak and worked with PHS MMU Deployment Teams 3 and 4. Even though some patients were admitted during my time as commander, I was also tasked with two additional responsibilities. The first was the development of an educational program to train Liberian providers to operate the MMU, or a similar facility, upon our departure." Teams 3 and 4 both worked hard and developed a great program much appreciated by the participants. The training program culminated in a public health summit attended by Vice Admiral Vivek Murthy, university students, survivors, and representatives of the Liberian MOH. "The second task was to develop a plan to decommission the MMU in preparation for its transfer to the MOH. Team 4 committed themselves to the task and did an exceptional job."

RADM Elizondo handed over his command to RADM Scott Giberson, which commenced the exit strategy for the response and decommissioning of the MMU. RADM Elizondo states, "It was one of most exciting experiences in uniform, and I will forever appreciate being entrusted to serve as commander of the Ebola response along with other health services officers."

"Health services officers strongly impacted the success of this mission. It was this category that developed and executed a cross-disciplinary train-the-trainer workshop in which other healthcare workers from outside ETUs, came to the MMU and trained with the Corps. Subsequently, MMU Corps officers also went to their ETUs and trained on site with them. Training was provided in everything from hand washing to the use of ultrasound to performance of CPR to resiliency. It was a four-day workshop for all healthcare workers and resulted in a certificate of completion with a graduation. It is the multidisciplinary nature of this category that lends us to be successful with a lot of the developing mission needs."

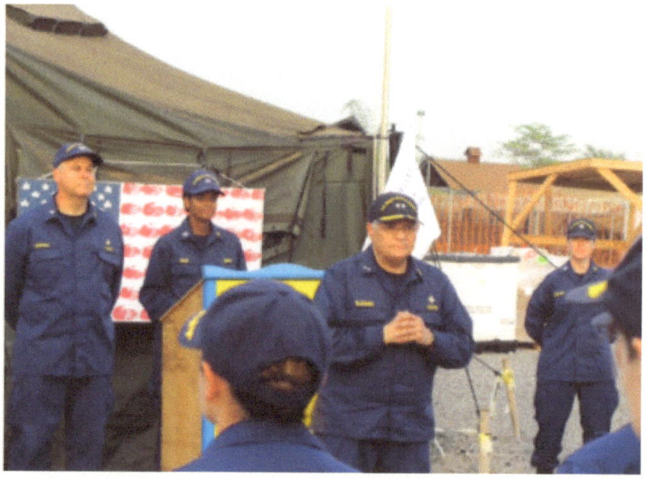

RADM Elizondo is seen here, hands clasped, speaking to the officers of the MMU under his command.

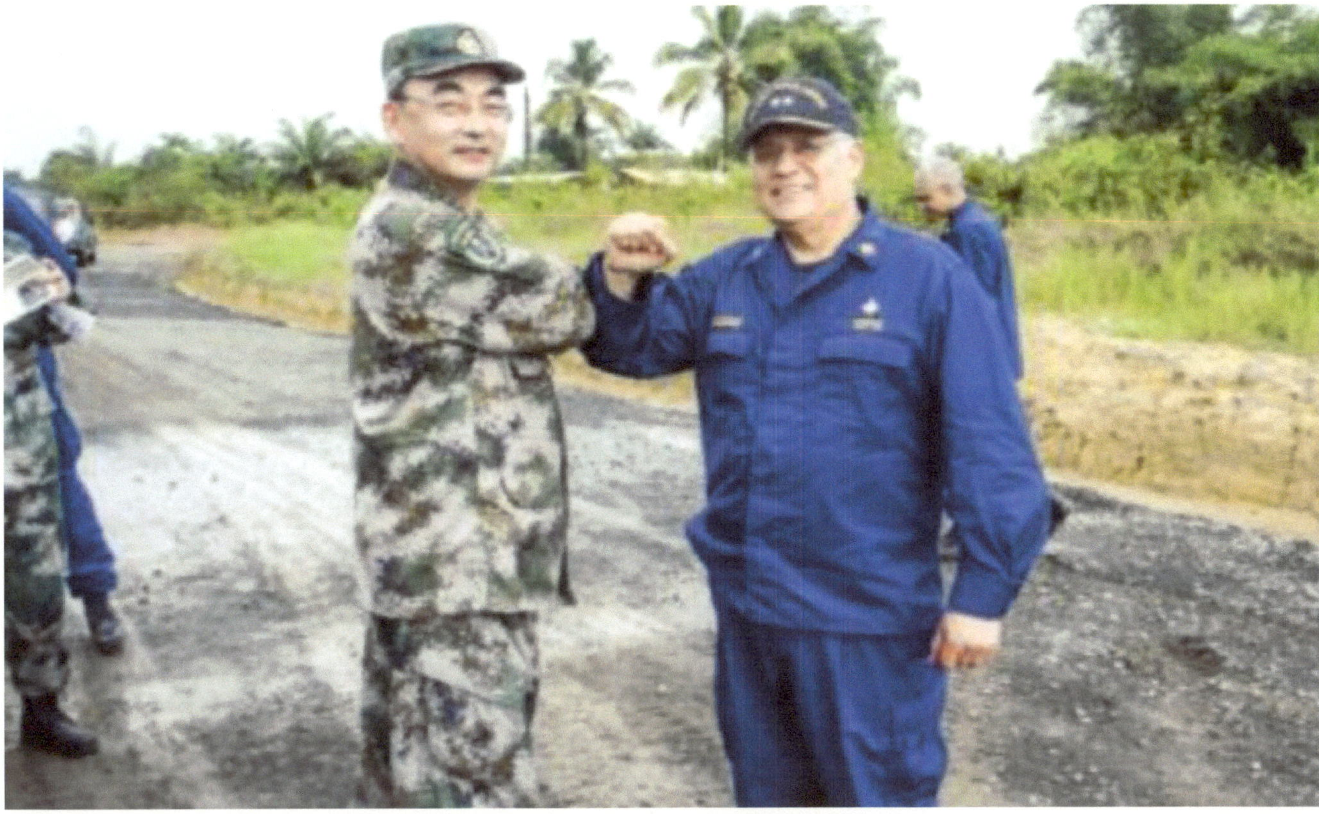

RADM Elizondo *(right)* and Senior Colonel Chunquan *(left)* exchange cordialities "MMU style."

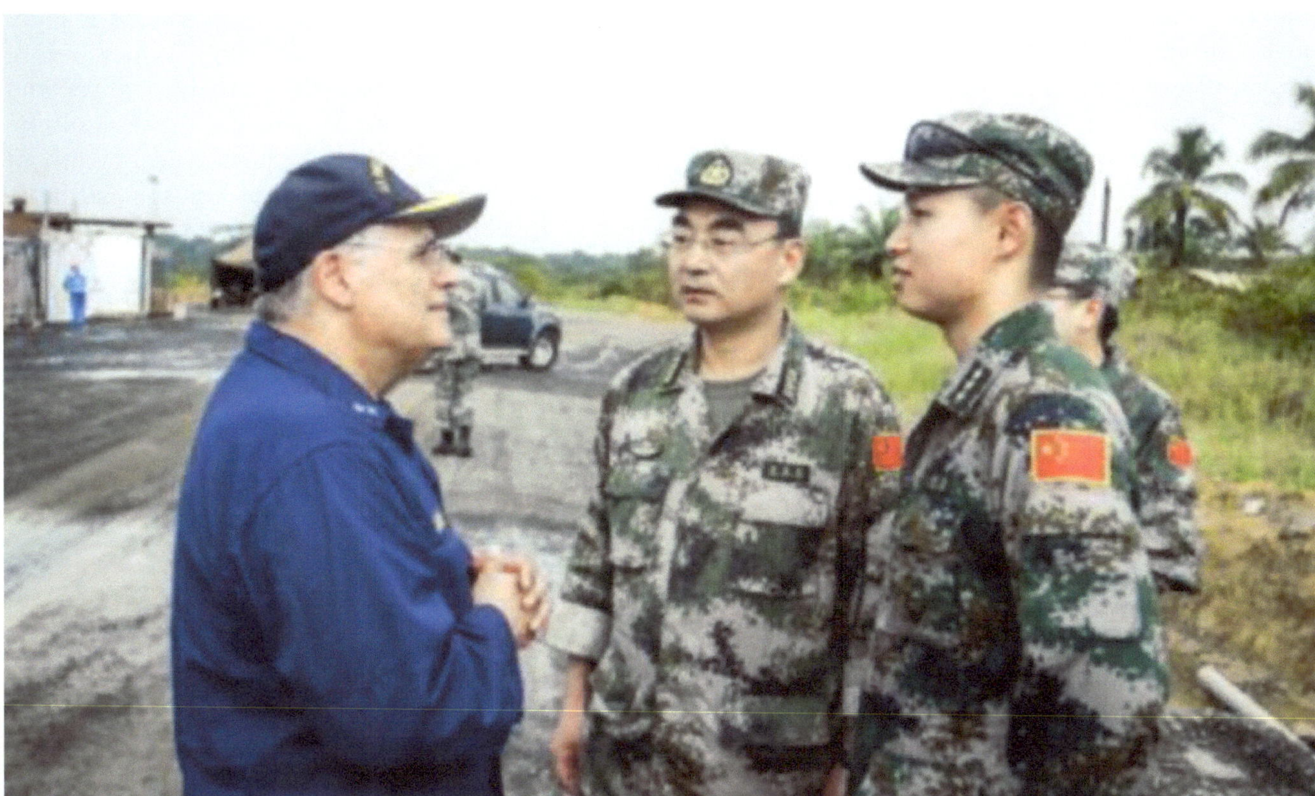

RADM Elizondo, Senior Colonel Chunquan, and CAPT Shen finish the MMU tour with a final assessment and appreciation of the services provided at the MMU.

CAPT David de la Cruz

"[I] will forever remember having watched dedicated and resilient officers rise to the occasion."

—David de la Cruz, PhD, MPH
DOIC and Executive Officer, MMU Team 2

CAPT David de la Cruz was humbled by the honor and privilege to have served as the Monrovia Medical Unit (MMU) Team 2's deputy Officer-in-Charge (DOIC) and executive officer. The MMU's mission was to provide care for both Liberian and international health care workers who had become infected with Ebola while caring for patients in Liberia. Being a part of MMU Team 2 provided him with the opportunity to serve alongside some of the best and brightest, not only in the United States Public Health Service (USPHS), but anywhere in the US government.

A group of seventy-six individual officers quickly bonded to become the best of the Public Health Service (PHS). The USPHS Commissioned Corps officers who came together to form MMU Team 2 began as individuals who were all committed to the same goal of providing compassionate, high-quality care. But before they left their training in Anniston, they had become a team of committed officers who were singularly focused on safely completing the mission.

While it can be argued that nobody could have been completely prepared for this deployment, CAPT de la Cruz was always confident in the Commissioned Corps officers' ability to succeed in completing the mission. He remains particularly proud of the junior officers on his team and those on their first deployment. Time and again, they stepped up and exceeded his high expectations. Each day presented MMU Team 2 with challenges and struggles. CAPT de la Cruz shared that he "will forever remember having watched dedicated and resilient officers rise to the occasion".

Successfully completing this mission without a significant safety incident and bringing all of his teammates home in good health remains a highlight of his USPHS career. Being a member of MMU Team 2 has made him a better officer and leader. CAPT de la Cruz will be forever grateful to his teammates, family, and the leadership of USPHS who made it possible for him to participate in this life-changing deployment.

MMU Team 2 built on excellence and finished strong!

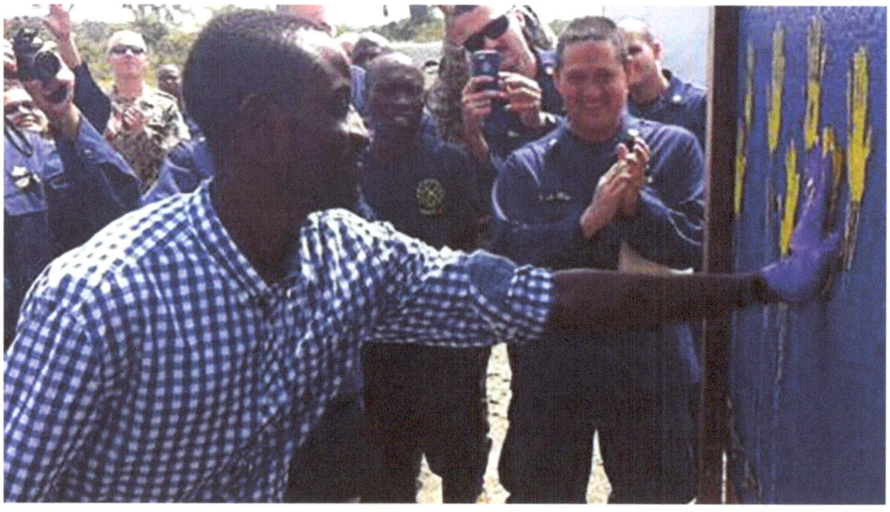

CAPT de la Cruz watches an MMU patient place his handprint on the MMU Survivor Wall during a ceremony.

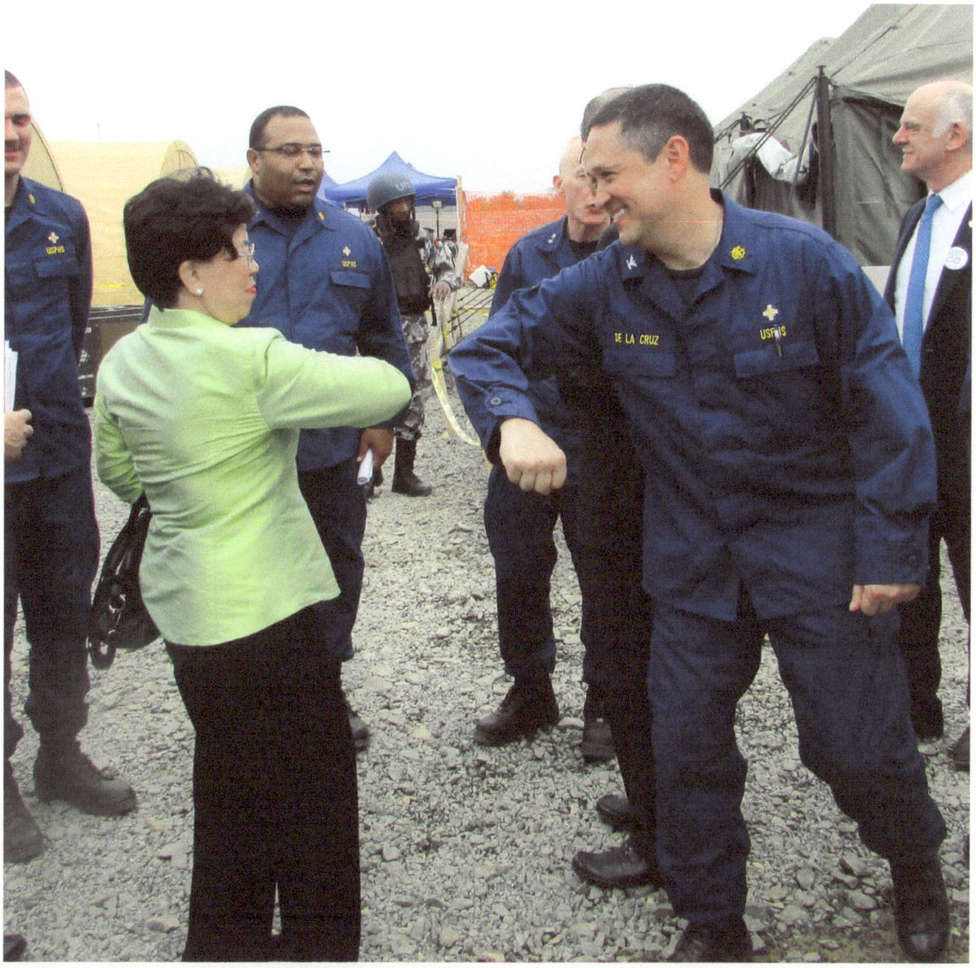

CAPT de la Cruz gives an elbow bump to then- World Health Organization (WHO) Director-General Margaret Chan during a tour of the MMU.

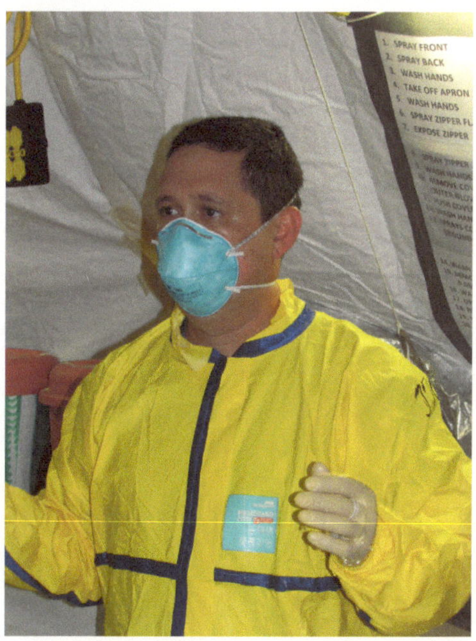

CAPT de la Cruz is fitted with personal protective equipment (PPE) at the MMU.

CAPT Robin MacGowan & LT Heather Joseph

Liberia Reintroduction Outbreak "Successfully Contained"

—Robin MacGowan, MPH and Heather Joseph, MPH

CAPT Robin MacGowan and LT Heather Joseph (Health Services category) were deployed to Monrovia, Liberia, from May to June 2015 as members of the Centers for Disease Control and Prevention (CDC) Liberia Epi Team, along with LCDR Lisa Belcher (Scientist category). These officers primarily served on the CDC Rapid Response Team and developed standard operating procedures (SOPs) for the immediate deployment of CDC staff should a re-introduction of Ebola Virus Disease (EVD) into Liberia occur. The Rapid Response Team's SOP outlines implementation of the Rapid Isolation and Treatment of Ebola strategy in Liberia in response to this potential threat. The officers also provided technical assistance to county health teams to develop county-specific plans in the event of a confirmed EVD case in Liberia. In late June 2015, following the departure of CAPT MacGowan, LT Joseph, and LCDR Belcher, their work in preparing for a reintroduction event served the CDC well, as it made an effective response to actual re-introduction of Ebola in Liberia—an outbreak that was successfully contained to only six cases with two deaths.

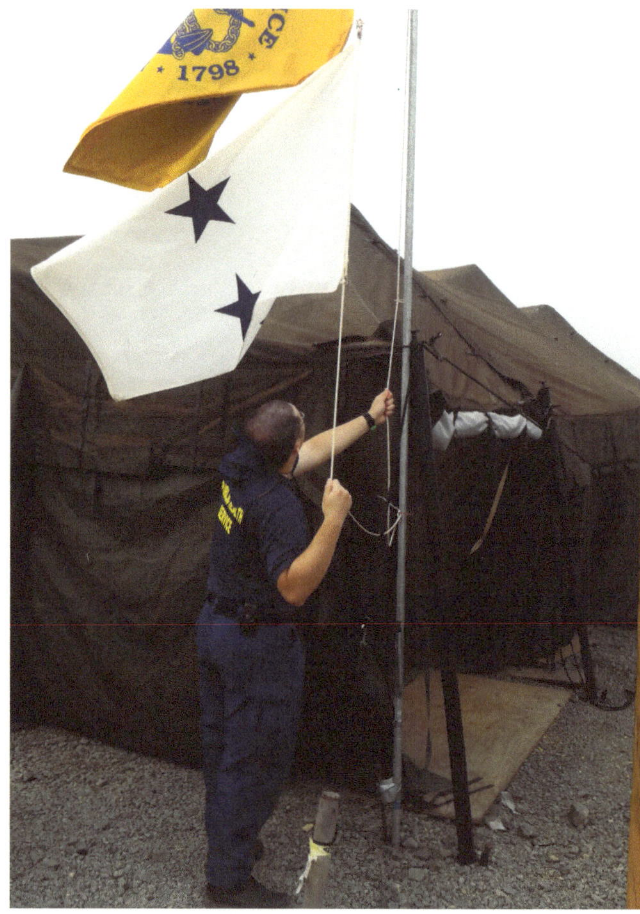

USPHS officers participate in daily raising and lowering of personal USPHS Commissioned Corps service flags over Camp Eason Monrovia Medical Unit (MMU). LCDR Yang raises USPHS Commissioned Corps and RADM Elizondo flags.

CAPT Cynthia Spells

"The members of my team became family . . ."

—Cynthia Spells, LCSW, MVF-CSW, ACSW, BCD

CAPT Cynthia Spells served as the chief behavioral health officer for Monrovia Medical Unit (MMU) Team 4 from March 1 to May 1, 2015. She shares, "This deployment was an experience of a lifetime. To be part of such a historical event will be something that I will never forget." She remembers that the people of Monrovia, Liberia, were grateful and appreciative of the United States Public Health Service (USPHS) presence and support. "They were in awe that we were willing to risk our own well-being to support them in their time of need." CAPT Spells believes that in this moment of world crisis, the Commissioned Corps really showed its value to the world. She explains, "The members of my team became family, and there will be an ongoing connection as a result of this shared experience."

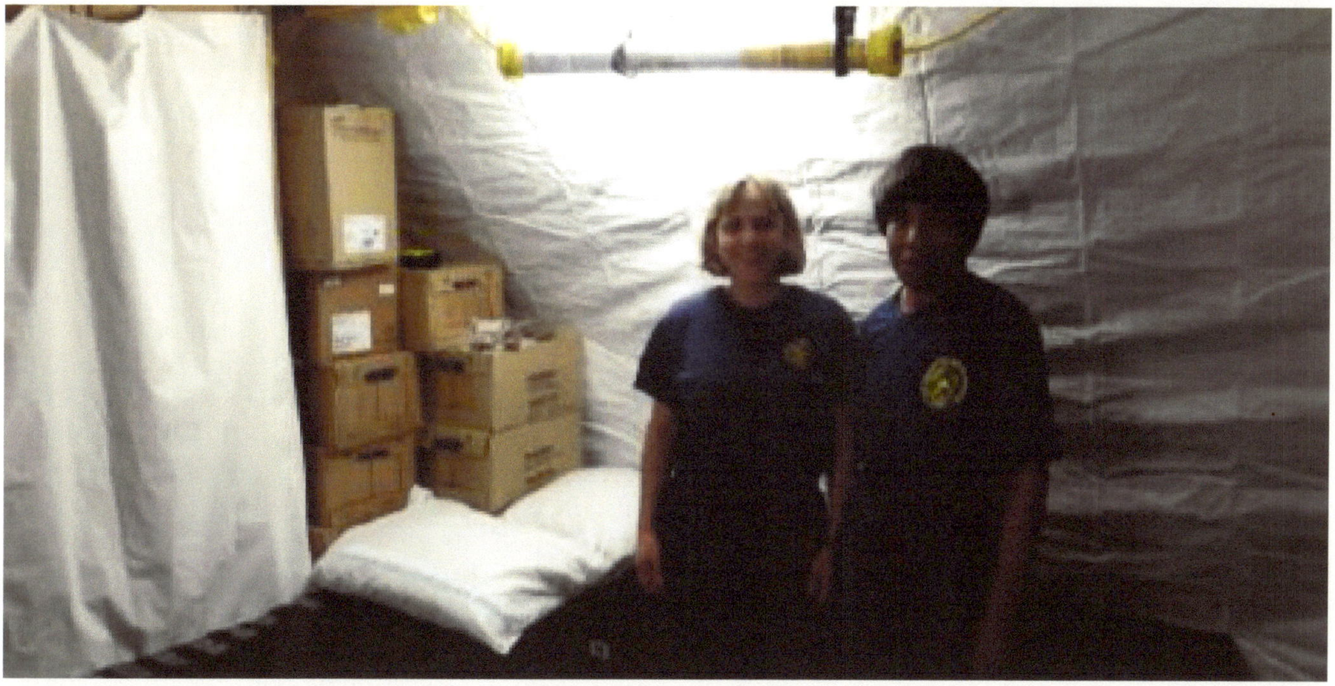

CAPT Spells *(right)* and CDR Fermin *(left)* are pictured in the behavioral health treatment area of Camp Eason's MMU. This section included several rest areas to allow MMU officers to decompress during shifts.

CAPT Robin Hunter Buskey

"To access villages, most days involved many hours traveling on muddy roads in a land cruiser and periodically involved extensive trekking with some travel via United States military and United Nations aircraft."

"I accepted this mission as part of my personal responsibility to combat disease worldwide and contribute to the reduced incidence and prevalence of Ebola."

—Robin Hunter Buskey, PA-C

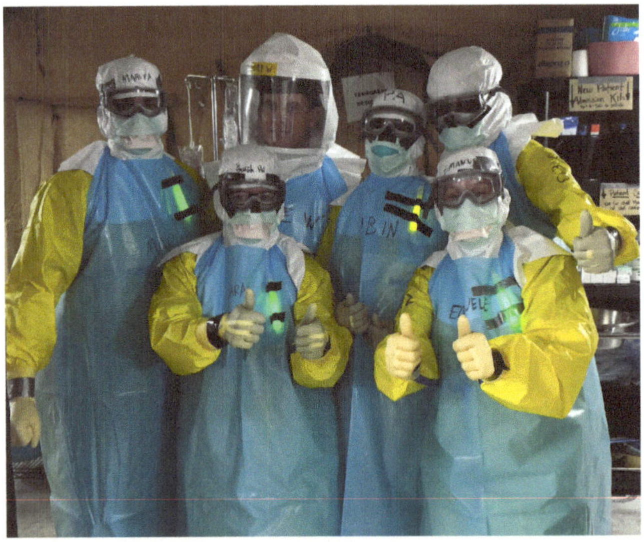

CAPT Buskey *(third from left, back row)* stands with the healthcare team in full personal protective equipment (PPE) at the MMU. Back Row: LCDR Maruna, LCDR Hickey, CAPT Buskey, CAPT Adams. Front row: LT Bailey, CDR Emanuele.

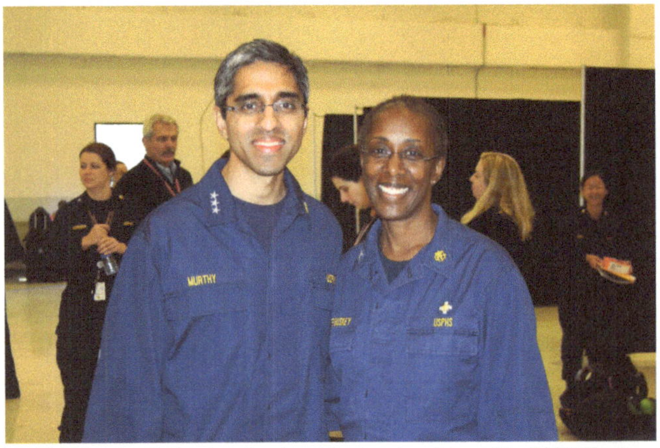

VADM Murthy *(left)* stands shoulder to shoulder with CAPT Buskey *(right)*.

CAPT Robin Buskey deployed in support of the Monrovia Medical Unit (MMU) as a medical house officer working with a team of physicians, physician assistants, and nurse practitioners. CAPT Buskey recalls, "I accepted this mission as part of my personal responsibility to combat disease worldwide and contribute to the reduced incidence and prevalence of Ebola. The key to controlling this epidemic was to stop it at its source in West Africa. That included providing support and care for those courageous healthcare workers and responders who were on the front lines combatting this disease." The focus of the MMU was to provide care to Liberian and international healthcare workers and responders who became infected with Ebola Virus Disease (EVD) and to expand capacity for responding and treating EVD. Healthcare workers and other Ebola responders were at higher risk of infection because of close sustained contact with Ebola patients who were symptomatic and infectious. The MMU received and provided care for many healthcare workers over six months. The Commissioned Corps' presence provided reassurance and created a safe environment for professionals who were working to combat EVD.

The team of specialized officers consisted of doctors, physician assistants, nurse practitioners, nurses, infection control officers, pharmacists, laboratorians, behavioral health specialists, and administrative management staff. The Commissioned Corps was the only US asset with direct patient care responsibilities.

"What I learned," CAPT Buskey explains, "was how to provide direct acute and ongoing care for patients suspected or confirmed to have the Ebola virus. I became an expert user of personal protective equipment (PPE). I developed enhanced diagnostic skills, as I could not use a stethoscope, my sense of touch, or smell for patient evaluation. A coordinated team effort was required to enter the high-risk zone. During my downtime, I practiced for the United States Public Health Service (USPHS) Music Ensemble concert later that year, exercised, danced, and enjoyed the phone calls and care packages from home."

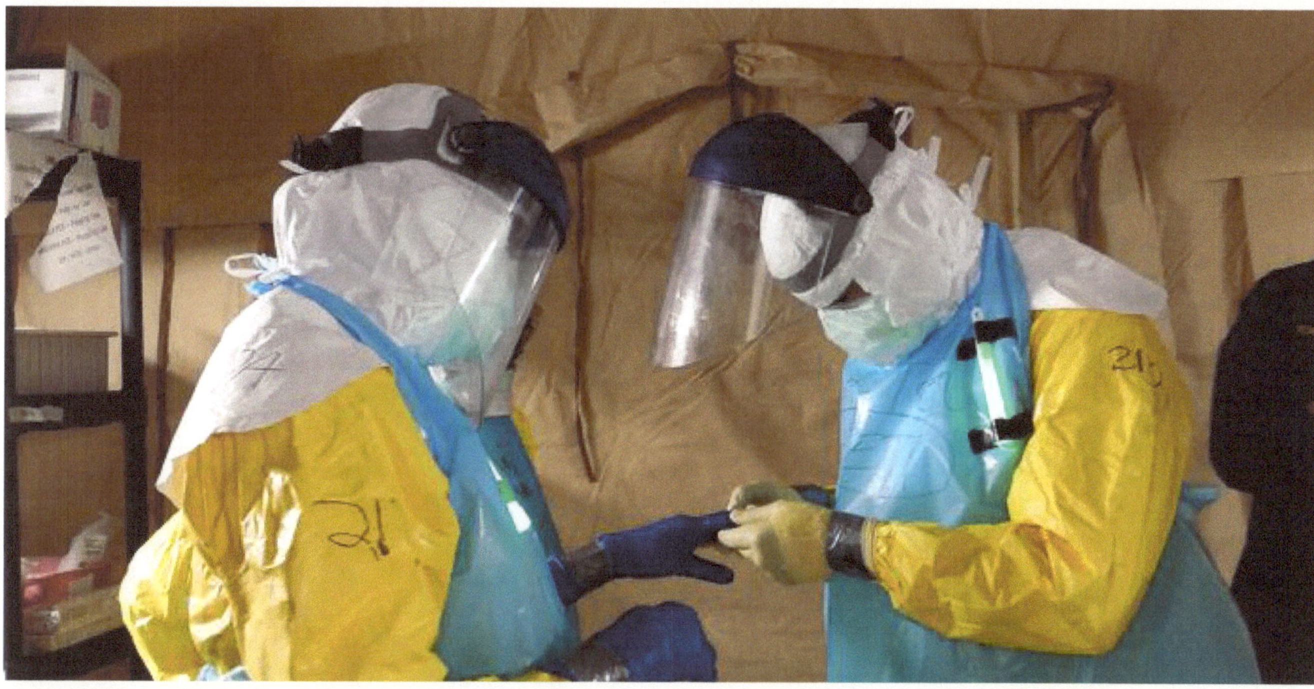

CAPT Buskey and LCDR Hickey examine each other's gloves for holes or tears to ensure that their PPE is fully intact.

CAPT Buskey goes on to say, "I am grateful to have contributed to the creation of Ebola clinical practice guidelines, staff and patient education, preparation of case summaries, and all of the medical services provided at the MMU. Additionally, I appreciate the genuine camaraderie and eternal bonds formed with my team."

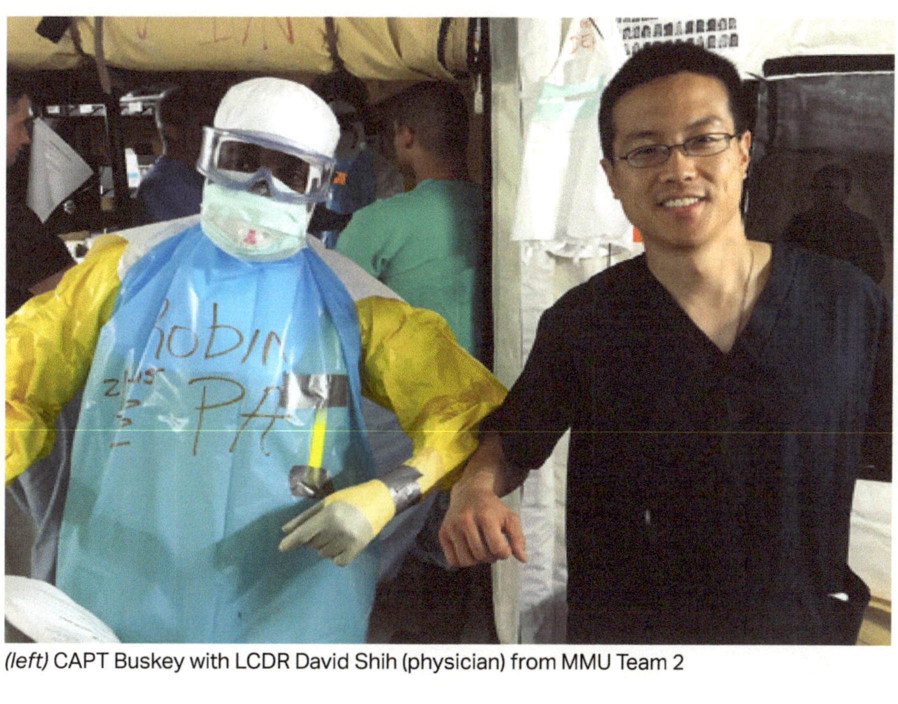

(left) CAPT Buskey with LCDR David Shih (physician) from MMU Team 2

CAPT (Ret.) Dorothy Stephens

"We were told that we were unique in that we had been culled from different agencies . . . and all spoke French at the near-native, if not native, level."

—Dorothy Stephens (Ret.)

CAPT Dorothy Stephens' permanent duty station was the Health Resources and Services Administration (HRSA). She was one of nine USPHS Commissioned Corps officers temporarily assigned to the Centers for Disease Control and Prevention (CDC) for the Ebola response in Guinea. CAPT Dorothy recalls, "We were told that we were unique in that we had been culled from different agencies, the Health Resources and Services Administration (HRSA), the Food and Drug Administration (FDA), the Substance Abuse and Mental Health Services Association (SAMHSA), the Department of Defense (DOD), the Office of the Secretary (OS), the Federal Bureau of Prisons (BOP), and the Indian Health Service (IHS), and all spoke French at the near-native, if not native, level.

"Four of our contingents spent a week in Anniston, Alabama, where they were trained in infection control and prevention. CAPT Andreason preceded us to Guinea and functioned as the team lead for the Border Health Team. The remaining eight met and bonded over a week in Atlanta, where we were trained in a myriad of Ebola and CDC logistical-related subjects. Prior to our departure, we were assigned tasks to assume in Guinea, however one of the most important lessons we learned was that we might go in as bakers but would could come out carpenters. In other words, we were to remain flexible."

As a team, much was accomplished. While CAPT Stephens managed the various projects funded through the CDC Foundation (a non-profit created by Congress to utilize private sector funding and services in support of the CDC's mission), other members of the team contributed significant accomplishments to the mission's success. LT Marc Eric Djassa Bi Kakou and LCDR Matilda Fienkeng trained healthcare workers in the Ebola endemic prefecture of Boffa. LT Viky Verna implemented a training project for religious leaders and body washers in the prefecture of Dubréka. LCDR Benoit Dagadu deployed epidemiologists up-country. LCDR Joseph Ndifor functioned as a case detection agent, and LCDR Michael Kluk worked on implementing health communications projects nationwide.

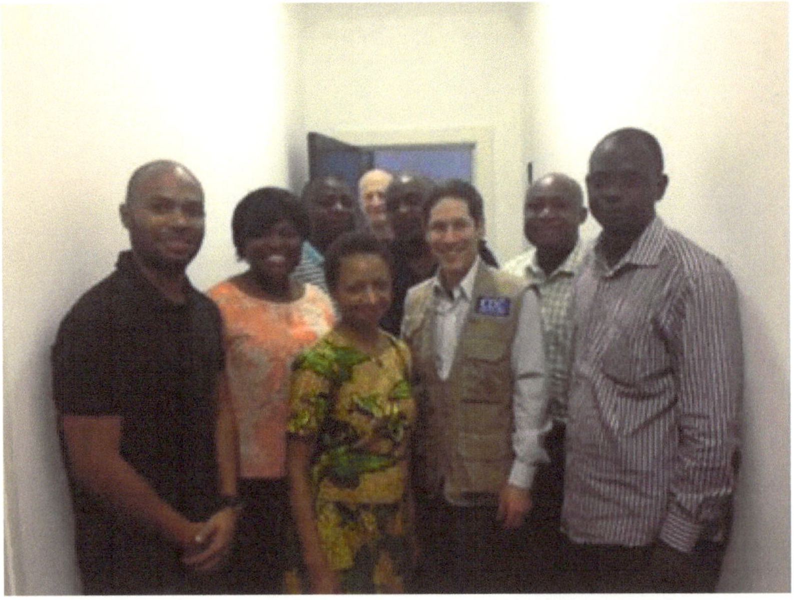

The team with CDC Director Dr. Tom Frieden. From left to right *(front row)* LT Vern; LCDR Fienkeng; CAPT Stephens; Dr. Frieden; and LCDR Dagadu. Back row: LT Djassa, CAPT Andreason, and LCDR Ndifor.

CAPT Robert Windom

"All the officers involved showed extreme flexibility, camaraderie, and compassion in meeting the global public health mission amidst the most austere and hazardous conditions."

—Robert Windom, MPH, MBA, CHES

In October 2014, CAPT Robert Windom was selected as a member of Team 1 deploying to staff Camp Eason, the twenty-five-bed Monrovia Medical Unit (MMU) field hospital. He says, "This was a humbling experience, to be one of the first sixty-nine officers to answer the call for this historic mission. I was called to fill a position on the Medical Records and Administration team, but I stepped up immediately to assist whenever and wherever needed." CAPT Windom assisted in areas such as planning, operations, and facility engineering. "I also stepped up in roles that were completely out of my normal comfort level, such as assisting the movement of deceased Ebola Virus Disease (EVD) patients," CAPT Windom shares. "I accepted this mission with a goal to make a positive difference and help diminish the threat of EVD by doing whatever was necessary for my team. All the officers involved showed extreme flexibility, camaraderie, and compassion in meeting the global public health mission amidst the most austere and hazardous conditions."

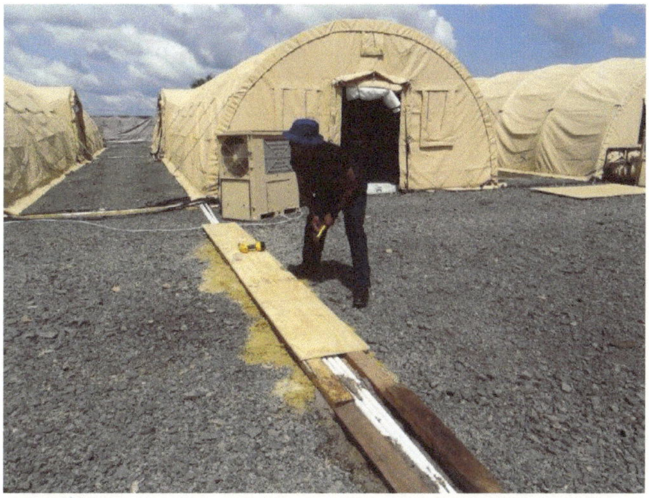

CAPT Windom does a bit of facility engineering, laying down raw plywood to protect pipes draining from one of the sand-colored MMU tents.

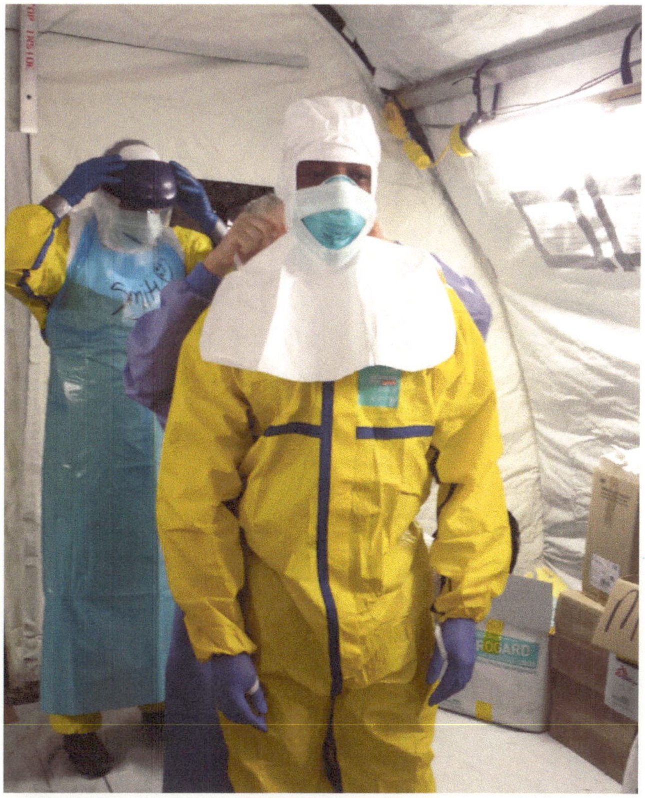

CAPT Windom dons personal protective equipment (PPE).

CAPT Michael Schmoyer

"My office was initially given authority to coordinate whole-of-government cooperation, communications, and collaboration . . ."

—Michael Schmoyer, PhD

In 2014, CAPT Michael Schmoyer was the director of the Office of Pandemics and Emerging Threats within the Health and Human Services' (HHS's) Office of Global Affairs (OGA). In May 2014, the National Security Council charged the OGA to coordinate the Washington, DC–based aspects of the Ebola response. (The Centers for Disease Control and Prevention [CDC] was responsible for coordinating efforts in Africa.) CAPT Schmoyer's team in the OGA coordinated the US government's efforts relating to the Ebola response in Washington, DC, from May until August, when the US Agency for International Development's (USAID's) Response Management Team was established. CAPT Schmoyer recalls, "My office was initially given authority to coordinate whole-of-government cooperation, communications, and collaboration until August. Once disasters were formally declared within the three stricken African countries, the United States Agency for International Development took on the coordination of both DC-based efforts and those in Africa."

In September 2014, President Obama approved the USPHS Commissioned Corps to deploy to Liberia to provide clinical care to healthcare workers afflicted with Ebola. CAPT Schmoyer worked with RADM Giberson and a handful of others to develop the concept of operations for the Monrovia Medical Unit (MMU). Then, early in October 2014, he deployed as part of the Advanced Echelon (ADVON) team, which prepared the MMU in advance of MMU Team 1. Major roles of the ADVON team included supporting the Department of Defense (DOD) in building the MMU, developing a tasking support system with USAID to provide logistical support to the forthcoming USPHS MMU teams and establishing onsite Ebola Treatment Unit (ETU) training programs for MMU staff with non-governmental organizations (NGOs) in Liberia. On his second deployment, CAPT Schmoyer worked as part of the Transition Team to stand down the MMU and transition the site to be run by the government of Liberia. He supported Embassy Monrovia with the transition of DOD/US African Command to DOD/101st Division as the supporting element for the MMU.

Currently, CAPT Schmoyer's team in HHS's Office of Security and Strategic Information is very involved with the National Security Council staff and other national security stakeholders addressing the 2018 Ebola outbreak in the eastern region of the Democratic Republic of Congo.

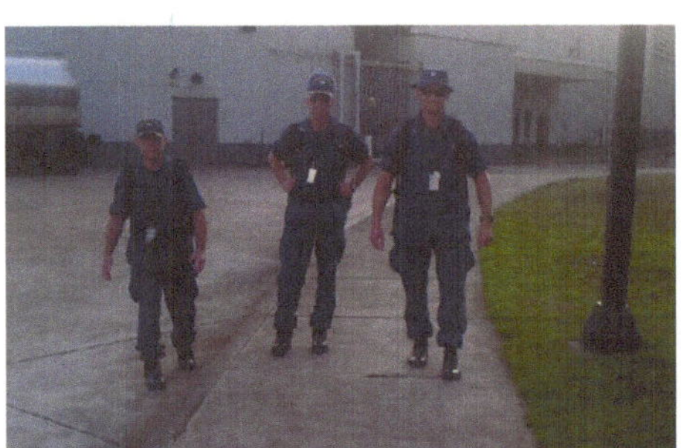

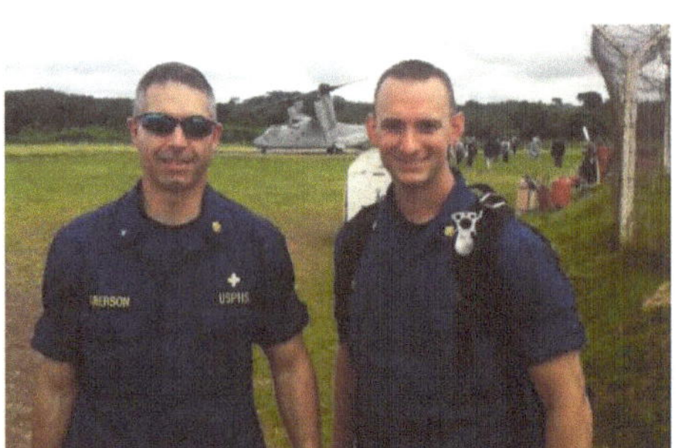

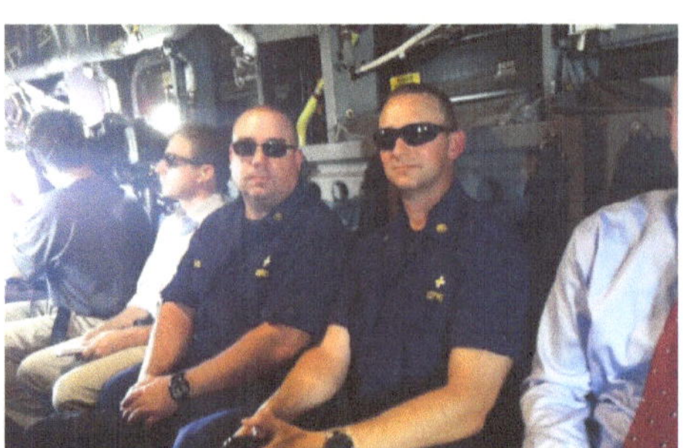

(far left) CAPT Bourg *(left)*, RADM Dieser *(middle)*, and CAPT Schmoyer *(right)* outside of Embassy Monrovia. *(middle)* RADM Giberson *(left)* and CAPT Schmoyer *(right)* are dropped off by an Osprey at an ETU in Liberia. *(far right)* CAPT Davis *(left)* and CAPT Schmoyer *(right)* ride aboard a US Marine Corps Osprey over Liberia.

CDR Kenneth Monahan

"The time investment by the field project officers for the work with Ebola Virus Disease is remarkable."

—Kenneth Monahan, FACHE, MHSA, EMT

CDR Monahan served as a field project officer and facilitated the planning process for the Region III Ebola Virus Disease (EVD) Continuity of Operations that started in mid-2015. The culmination of this effort was the Table Top Exercise, which included over 120 federal, state, and local partners from throughout the six Region III states. The Office of the Assistant Secretary for Preparedness and Response (ASPR) Hospital Preparedness Program (HPP) provides healthcare-focused funding to sixty-two awardees: fifty states, three large municipalities, and nine[5] US territories. The HPP was chosen as a vehicle to disperse Ebola funding to the sixty-two awardees. This was due to heightened awareness and risk of Ebola and to prepare the nation to receive patients with EVD. The funding was available in two parts: Part A was distributed among all of the awardees and totaled $162 million. Part B totaled $32.5 million for the development of ten Ebola Treatment Centers (ETCs) located at regional hospitals across the United States. The awardees were required to complete applications to request appropriate funding. CDR Monahan shares, "The HPP field project officers (FPOs) like myself provided a critical link between the national program and awardees. Beginning in October 2014, the FPOs were directly involved with the Rapid Ebola Preparedness team visits and assessment visits to hospitals. In addition, there were other Ebola-related activities that the HPP and the FPOs were involved in daily when the first American Ebola patient arrived in the United States for treatment in August 2014. Each of the FPOs provided countless hours facilitating the application process for sixty-two awardees." This included reviewing applications, reviewing finance, tracking major funding categories, meeting with awardees and grant managers in person and over the phone, providing technical assistance, and meeting with regional partners to inform them of developments. CDR Monaghan believes that Ebola-related activities will continue for several years. FPOs will be participating in ongoing training for the regional ETCs' visits to the National Ebola Training and Education Center. In addition, FPOs in each region are facilitating the development of transportation and operation plans for Ebola and other special pathogens. These plans comprise essential elements of the course of care for an Ebola patient. CDR Monahan states, "The time investment by the field project officers for the work with Ebola Virus Disease is remarkable. The time spent with these duties does not take into account the normal steady-state activities and work requirements that the FPOs do on a daily basis, which also includes response operations and deployments, like hurricane response or National Special Security Events." He adds, "In April 2018, the Tranquil Terminus exercise was completed. This exercise was a cooperative effort between the Health and Human Services (HHS) and the Department of State and is the largest full-scale exercise that HHS has ever conducted. ASPR Regional Coordinators and FPOs in Regions 4, 6, 9, and 10 participated to provide communication and coordination to move patients from assessment hospitals to regional ETCs."

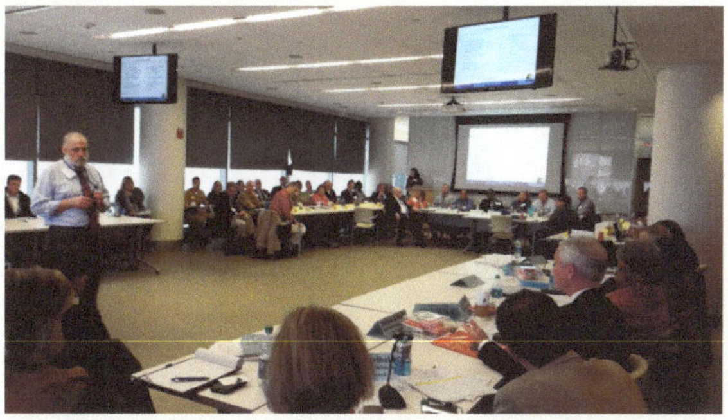

Table Top Exercise occurred in April 2018 at the Johns Hopkins Hospital in Baltimore. Hopkins is the Region III ETC.

5—https://www.federalgrantswire.com/hospital-preparedness-program-hpp-ebola-preparedness-and-response-activities.html#.XTie_02P6Uk

CDR Joseph Roth Jr.

"To access villages, most days involved many hours traveling on muddy roads in a land cruiser and periodically involved extensive trekking with some travel via United States military and United Nations aircraft."

—Joseph Roth Jr, MPH

CDR Joseph Roth Jr. was deployed to Liberia from October to November 2014, during the height of the Ebola outbreak. During that period, CDR Roth worked in six rural counties to conduct contact tracing, identify new cases, and build epidemiologic capacity. Based primarily in southeast Liberia, his deployment often involved working in remote villages, some with known Ebola transmission, while performing a spectrum of duties that included building epidemiology capacity, educating health staff and community members, interviewing household members of patients, transporting specimens, examining construction of community care centers in villages and a refugee camp, and negotiating transport of suspected and probable cases. He says, "To access villages, most days involved many hours traveling on muddy roads in a land cruiser and periodically involved extensive trekking with some travel via United States military and United Nations aircraft. During one mission, my team was flown on a Blackhawk by the 101st Airborne Division and dropped off at a remote village to collect specimens where Ebola was circulating. As there were no roads near the village, our return entailed hiring local guides to lead an hours-long trek and crossing a river by dugout canoe in order to arrange pickup by a Peace Corps vehicle." Working under taxing circumstances was, at times, quite challenging. However, CDR Roth explains, "My team was able to have a positive impact, and I am thankful to have had an opportunity to contribute to the mission."

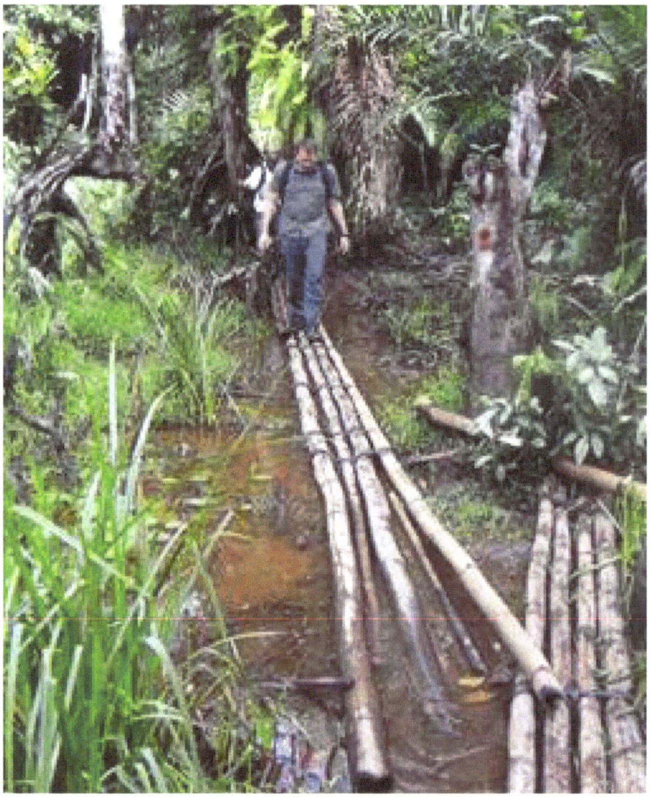

CDR Roth walks across sodden, muddy ground to access remote villages where Ebola virus disease (EVD) was circulating.

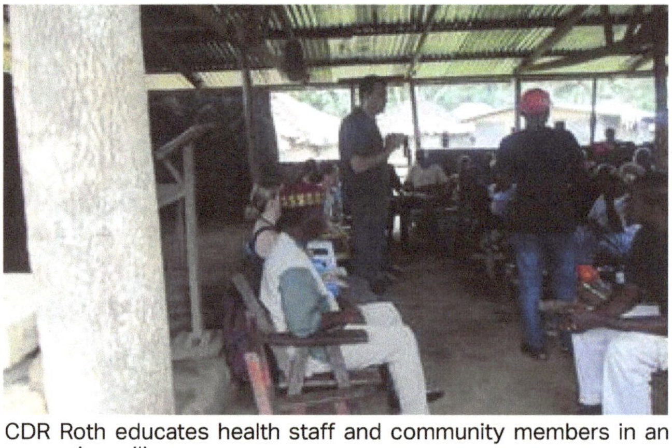

CDR Roth educates health staff and community members in an open-air pavilion.

CDR Charlene Majersky

"The aspect most meaningful to me was building an efficient, productive, and spirited team during the Centers for Disease Control and Prevention (CDC)'s largest international response . . ."

—Charlene Majersky, PhD, MPH

CDR Charlene Majersky served as the Ebola Program management officer for the Centers for Disease Control and Prevention (CDC)'s Division of Global Migration and Quarantine (DGMQ) and team lead of the Ebola Coordination Team for the Quarantine and Border Health Services Branch. She shares, "I stood up and led an Ebola response coordination team, which managed finance and administrative initiatives to support the DGMQ, Global Migration Task Force, and the Quarantine and Border Health Services Branch. The aspect most meaningful to me was building an efficient, productive, and spirited team during the CDC's largest international response, which exhibited sound technical competence, excellent customer service, team cohesiveness, and a spirit to serve with heart!"

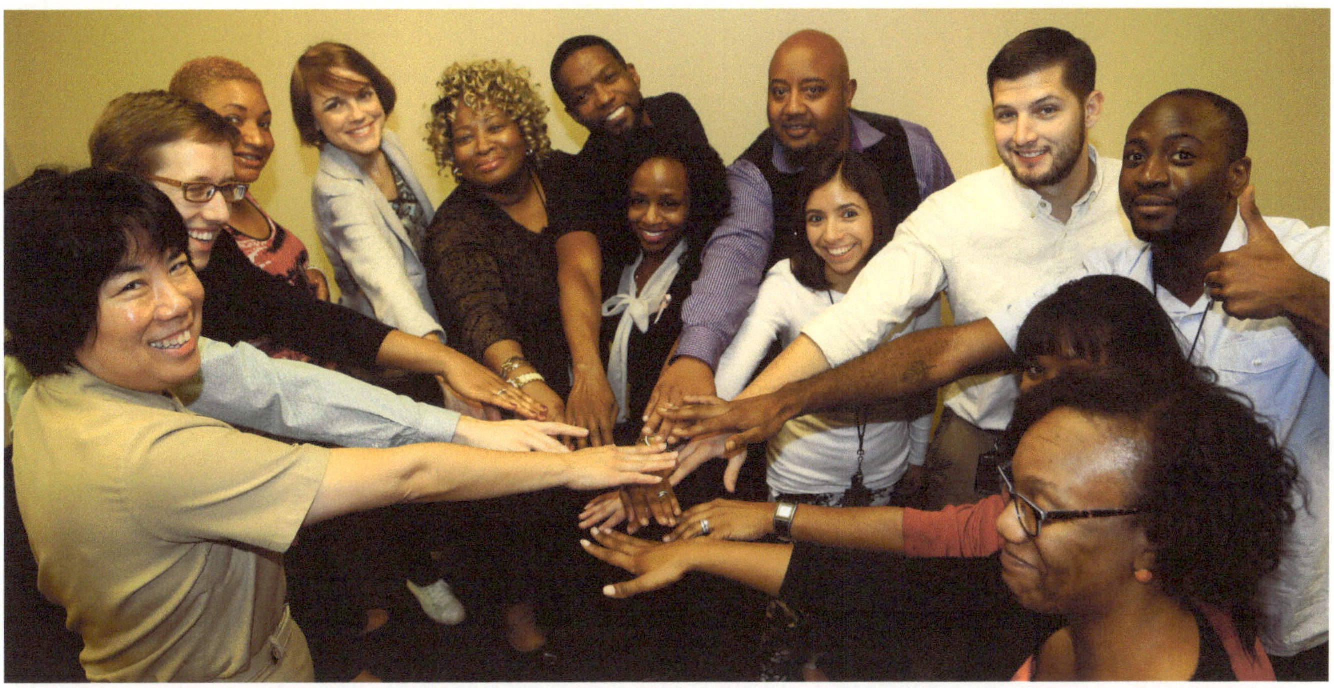

CDR Majersky *(bottom left)* is pictured with the robust team of CDC financial and management experts that supported the massive response effort of the agency.

CDR Torris Smith

"[We] were especially honored to support our United States Public Health Service (USPHS) colleagues by providing their families with . . . reunification tips upon the return of their family members to the United States."

—Torris Smith, MSW, LCSW, BCD

CDR Torris Smith and LCDR Arlin Hatch provided post-deployment support for families of Monrovia Medical Unit (MMU) Teams 3 and 4 in response to the Ebola epidemic. Improving the resiliency of the family was an important factor to consider for the reunification of the family after a deployment of this magnitude. Officers serving on this deployment encountered a swiftly growing outbreak that overwhelmed the healthcare infrastructure in the region. Rapidly shifting needs and priorities meant that officers often learned the specifics of their assignments only after arriving in their destination country. They were deployed to densely-populated urban centers, remote villages reachable only by foot, and everywhere in between. They left behind concerned loved ones for months at a time with limited communication. CDR Smith and LCDR Hatch "were especially honored to support our United States Public Health Service (USPHS) colleagues by providing their families with support, resiliency education, and reunification tips upon the return of their family members to the United States."

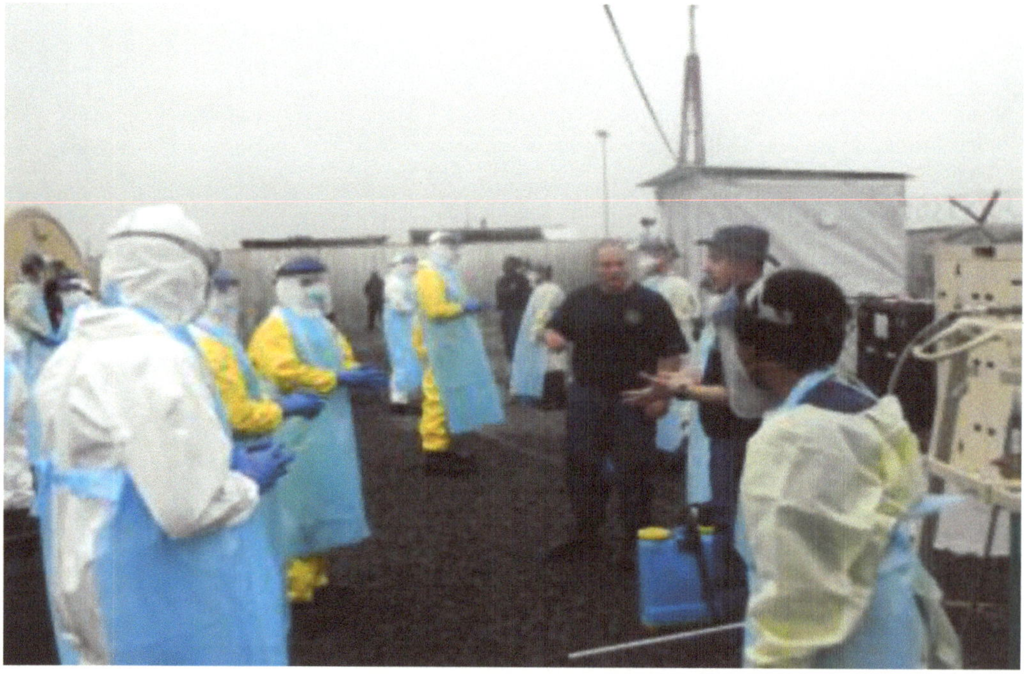

Camp Eason: Monrovia Medical Unit (MMU) Ebola Treatment Unit (ETU), Margibi County, Monrovia.

CDR Tobey Manns Royal

"This experience sincerely warmed my heart—not only seeing the appreciation but also hearing it from both deployed and returning officers and their family members."

—Tobey Manns Royal, MBA, MHA

CDR Tobey Manns-Royal deployed as a Family Support Network (FSN) administrative officer in the Secretary's Operations Center in Washington, DC, from February to May 2015. She provided support to families of officers deployed in response to Operation United Assistance at the Monrovia Medical Unit (MMU). CDR Manns-Royal was responsible for coordination of and participation in regular meetings with mental health teams, case managers, volunteers, and service access teams. She maintained and disseminated all media relations, including newsletters, emails, and Speaker Series presentations. She also managed data collection related to family and volunteers for regular reports. Her responsibilities resulted in a centralized service delivery, increased continuity of care and support to family members, increased accountability, increased customer service, and standardized information sharing.

As a part of this FSN administrator role, CDR Manns-Royal's responsibilities included conducting reintegration presentations that took place after officers returned from deployment but before they reunited with family. This allowed time for the returning officers to become familiar with the duties and responsibilities of the FSN and the assistance and support that was provided to their families while they were away. Officers were quick to share how they valued the additional support from the United States Public Health Service (USPHS) during their absence. CDR Manns-Royal says, "Serving as FSN administrator was truly an honor and privilege. This experience sincerely warmed my heart—not only seeing the appreciation but also hearing it from both deployed and returning officers and their family members. Knowing that family members of deployed officers are likely to experience some level of stress related to the deployment, my role in this response added to the collective skills to handle individuals in crisis."

The FSN supported deployed USPHS Commissioned officers, too. Whether their deployment lasted two weeks or a few months, the FSN connected families with a non-deployed state-side officer who would provide care coordination and wellness support. CDR Manns-Royal assisted in connecting the families of deployed officers with these PHS officers. This gave families a "listening ear" as well as the opportunity to connect with support options in their community. The FSN also provided families with additional assistance like shopping, arts and crafts, outdoor activities, event organization, PHS officer visits, food preparation, and driving.

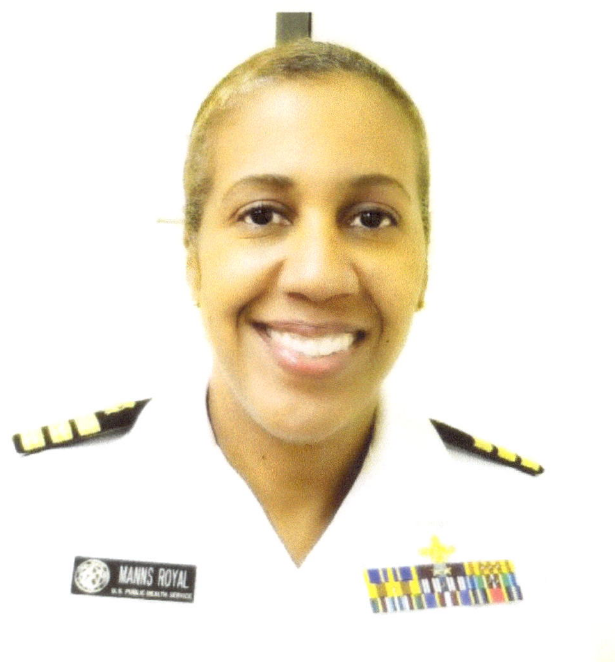

CDR Manns-Royal, USPHS, Health and Human Services (HHS), Bureau of Primary Health Care/Office of Quality Improvement.

CDRs Julie Chodacki and M. Sonsy Fermin

"We had an awesome opportunity to witness the resilience of the people of Liberia."

—Julie Chodacki, PsyD and M. Sonsy Fermin, LCSW

CDRs Julie Chodacki and M. Sonsy Fermin served as the Monrovia Medical Unit (MMU) Team 4 behavioral health providers. They recall, "We had an awesome opportunity to witness the resilience of the people of Liberia." After providing behavioral health support to Ebola patients and MMU Team 4 members during the initial phase of deployment, the commanders delivered training to Liberian healthcare providers who led the fight against Ebola. CDRs Chodacki and Fermin were struck that at the peak of the epidemic, the Liberian healthcare workers willingly placed their own lives in danger. In many cases, the Liberian workers were not paid as promised for their work, yet somehow they managed to maintain hope and gratitude. "It was hard to imagine that the Liberians wanted to learn from us, given that we learned so much from their example."

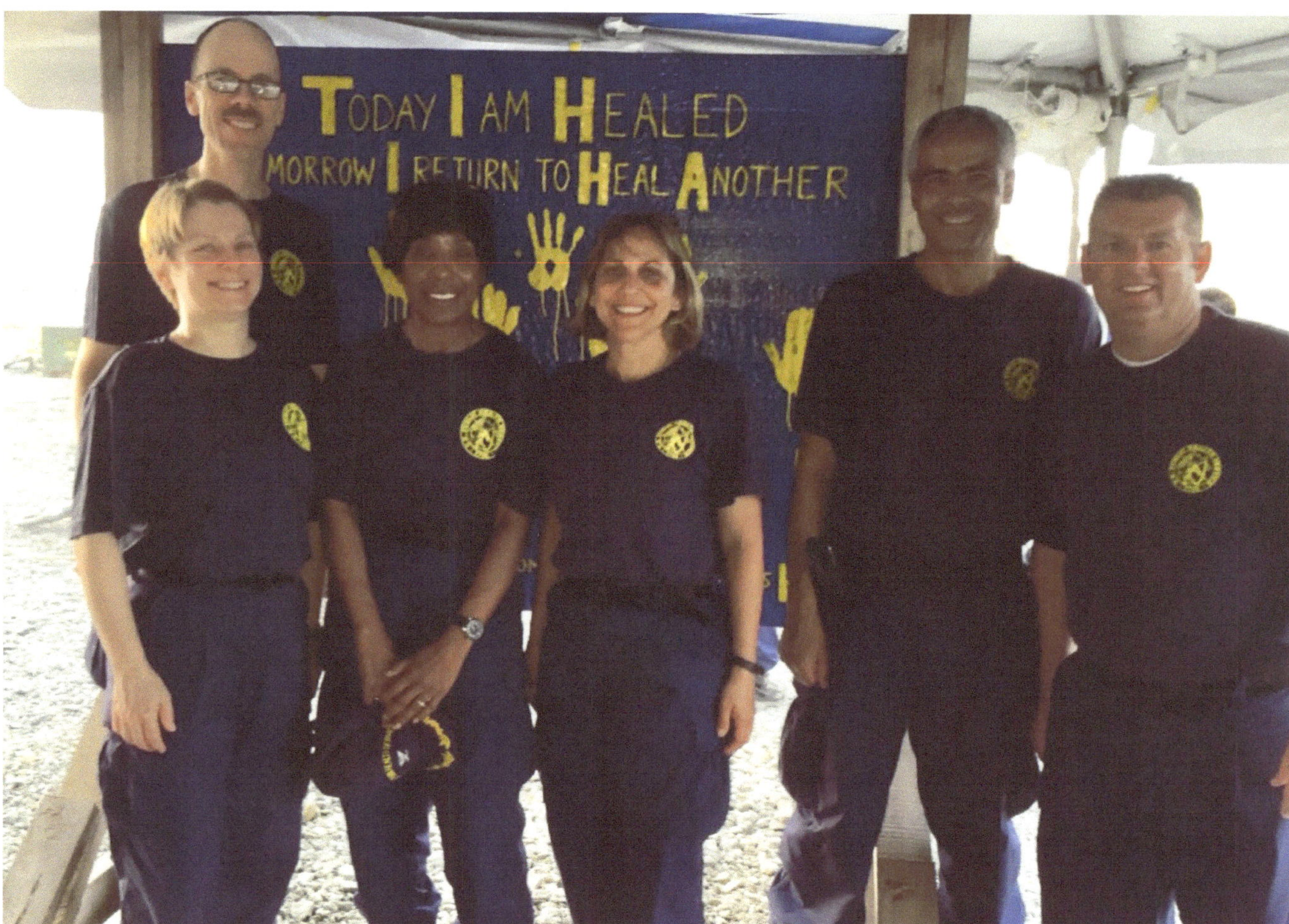

CDRs Chodacki (*front, far left*) and Fermin (*middle*) are pictured with members of the MMU Team 4 Mental Health Team.

CDR Andrew Chen

"Team 3 left in the wee hours of the night, and our first patient arrived that morning—no practice, no warmup, no help; we were on our own, and this was not a drill."

—Andrew Chen, MPH, MBA, FACHE, CEM

CDR Andrew Chen served as deputy Officer-in-Charge (DOIC) of Monrovia Medical Unit (MMU) Team 4, which was deployed to Harbel, Liberia. Led by RADM (then-CAPT) Jose Belardo (Ret.), our goal was to leave behind a legacy of hope by ensuring that local healthcare workers had the training they needed to sustain this fight against Ebola, as well as transitioning the patient-care mission of the MMU to the Liberian Ministry of Health (MOH). CDR Chen recounts, "I wound up as the DOIC purely by circumstance. I was originally supposed to be the logistics chief (and then the operations chief), but a last-minute scrub by the officer who was originally rostered as the DOIC left a void, and the decision-makers decided that I would make a good DOIC. I will say that it was a bit surreal to essentially be running a hospital again and in an Air Force field hospital, no less (in which I had trained back in June 2004 at Fort Drum, New York, but that's a different story for a different day)." Team 4 started off with a bang, arriving in Liberia to a patient census of zero at the MMU. But only four days after arriving in-country, they were notified that the unit would be receiving a confirmed Ebola-positive patient the next day. CDR Chen shares, "Team 3 left in the wee hours of the night, and our first patient arrived that morning—no practice, no warmup, no help; we were on our own, and this was not a drill. Our clinical and safety teams were absolutely brilliant—they took dive after dive, donning personal protective equipment (PPE) and going into the hot zone, doing their best to save the life of our patient while also protecting themselves and each other. I also got in on the action: I was cross-trained as a doffer. The doffer coaches the diver on how to remove PPE and sprays the diver down with a chlorine solution to break down and kill the Ebola virus. I spent as much as a full half-hour helping each diver get out of his or her protective gear." Sadly, their best efforts were all for naught; their patient passed away on the sixth day she was with them.

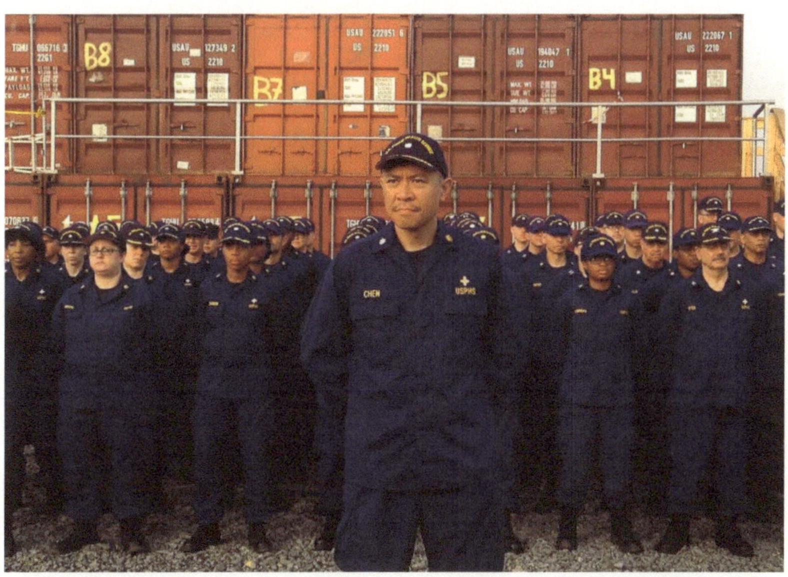

CDR Chen and the officers of MMU Team 4 stand at parade rest during the relief-in-place ceremony on March 20, 2015, taking over operations of the MMU from Team 3. Photo courtesy of the Office of US Foreign Disaster Assistance, United States Agency for International Development (USAID).

The team was able to conduct exchange visits with other Ebola Treatment Units (ETUs) in the greater Monrovia area. During these exchanges, there were opportunities to see the Liberian countryside. CDR Chen shares, "I have to admit, this is one of the poorest nations I've ever been in. The main highway that connects Monrovia (the country's capitol) with the international airport (which is near where we were located) is basically a small, two-lane road. There are small shops all along the road selling fish, cold drinks, sometimes groceries, wood carvings, and other sorts of knick-knack things. I've read that Liberia was on an economic upswing prior to the Ebola outbreak, after so many years of economic depression due to the civil wars and all, but early in the deployment most of the people I saw on the streets had a sort of resigned, fatalistic air about them as if this was their lot, and they would simply deal with it. If I take absolutely nothing else away from this deployment, the one thing I will take away is how good we have it in the United States, and how grateful I am for all the opportunities that we have. The term 'first world problem(s)' has taken on a completely new meaning for me."

By the time Team 4 left, though, he noticed a change in attitude. "More people were starting to smile, schools were open again, and I even saw kids playing soccer with glee on their faces. We also had the opportunity to invite a Liberian cultural troupe to come and perform for us, and it was a great experience to see how they sing and dance. As opposed to the sense of resignation I saw in the countryside, the dancers were all smiles and energetic it was good to see some sense of happiness returning to the people."

"If I take absolutely nothing else away from this deployment, the one thing I will take away is how good we have it in the United States, and how grateful I am for all the opportunities that we have. The term 'first world problem(s)' has taken on a completely new meaning for me."

—*CDR Andrew Chen*

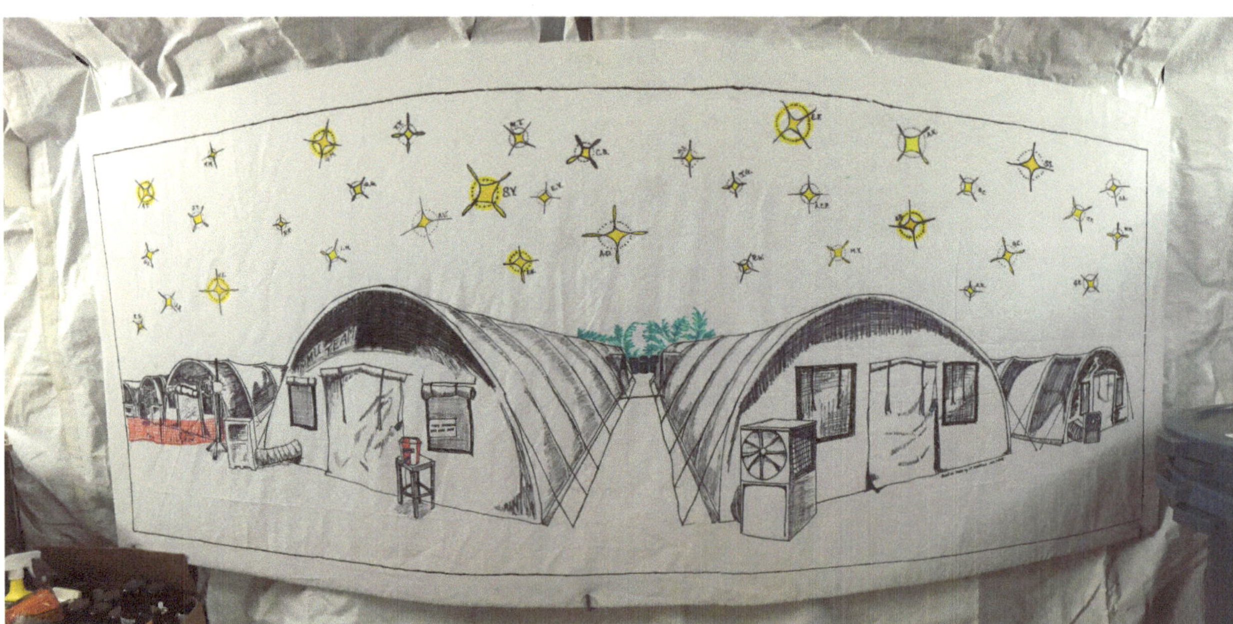

This mural, displayed inside the MMU, was created by CDR Peng and LCDR Wong. The mural depicts the tents of the camp, featuring the containment unit. There is a field of brilliant yellow stars above. Each star represents an MMU patient, the stars with the yellow halos represent a life claimed by the virus.

CDR Erich Kleinschmidt

"It was a mission that I was proud to be a part of and was certainly one of the highlights of my Public Health Service (PHS) career."

—Erich Kleinschmidt, MSW

CDR Erich Kleinschmidt was the team commander for Services Access Team (SAT) 5. He was deployed as part of the Reintegration Specialist mission to conduct Ebola symptom monitoring and case management as well as psycho-social support for the returning officers. All five SATs were deployed over the course of six months to support the return of public health officers from their deployment to Liberia. Each SAT included officers from a number of healthcare disciplines, including nurses, social workers, pharmacists, dieticians, healthcare administration, psychologists, and masters of public health. SAT officers were known as reintegration specialists. As part of their mission, each SAT facilitated a three-day team decompression upon return to the US, conducting twenty-one days of Ebola symptom monitoring in conjunction with the Centers for Disease Control and Prevention (CDC) and state health departments, and provided psycho-social support to address reintegration issues after the lengthy and austere deployment. The five SATs served over 230 officers over the course of five months.

CDR Kleinschmidt states, "It was personally quite gratifying to be involved in the Reintegration Specialist mission, as we were helping our own. These officers had deployed into life-threating circumstances, and we were there to support in any way we could to transition back to life stateside. The returning officers were understandably exhausted and slowly shifting their focus from treating patients and being on guard day and night against a deadly disease to normal living without fear of Ebola. Our reintegration specialists were responsible for monitoring and reporting the symptom checks to returned officer's respective state health departments. They also worked out arrangements between states, if an officer (under the 21 day monitoring window) needed to travel to another jurisdiction for a funeral or to visit a loved one. Our specialists were glad to be able to assist our officers in this capacity so they weren't burdened by the complexities of those arrangements. Our team did a great job supporting and encouraging while officers went through the twenty-one-day monitoring period and beyond. It was a mission that I was proud to be a part of and was certainly one of the highlights of my Public Health Service (PHS) career."

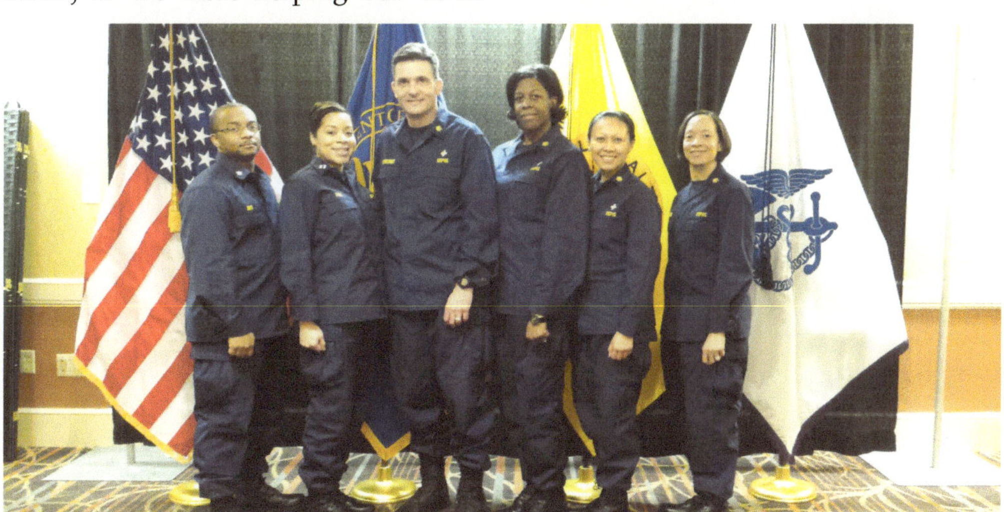

CDR Kleinschmidt *(middle)* poses with his team of reintegration specialists.

CDR Anthony Garza

"The Food and Drug Administration (FDA) Ebola Response Team was crucial . . . and exemplified the extraordinary dedication to the FDA mission and the public health of this nation."

—Anthony Garza, MS

CDR Anthony Garza was the Food and Drug Administration (FDA) lead responsible for tracking and reporting on the medical countermeasures (MCM) development activities in response to the Ebola outbreak in West Africa. CDR Garza explains, "The FDA's 2014 Ebola Response Team was established August 4, 2014, in response to Dr. Kent Brantly's arrival at Emory University for treatment after being diagnosed with Ebola virus disease." The Ebola Response Team was comprised of senior officials and subject-matter experts, both civilians and Commissioned Corps officers, from the various medical product centers and offices of the FDA. At the time of the outbreak, there were no current approved or licensed medical products for treatment, prevention, or diagnosis of Ebola virus. The FDA was asked to help expedite the development and availability of investigational medical products, including treatments, vaccines, diagnostic tests, and personal protective equipment (PPE). CDR Garza explains, "The main focus of the FDA's Ebola response had been to help provide scientific and regulatory advice to commercial developers and United States government agencies that support medical product development, including the National Institutes of Health (NIH), the Office of the Assistant Secretary for Preparedness and Response (ASPR), the Centers for Disease Control and Prevention (CDC), and the Department of Defense (DOD). The advice that the FDA provided helped to accelerate product development programs."

CDR Garza shares that he was originally contacted to deploy with Monrovia Medical Unit (MMU) Team 1 as a laboratorian but was unable to deploy due to being deemed mission critical for the FDA. "I was asked to serve as the lead response coordinator for the FDA tracking and reporting for the FDA Ebola Response Team. I reported on the MCM development activities in response to the Ebola outbreak in West Africa. I was able to produce 121 agency situation reports that provided the daily updates for the commissioner and her senior staff. These reports provided the input for the daily updates sent to the secretary and were used in the development and planning of the interagency response. As a member of this FDA Ebola Response Team, I actively worked with federal colleagues, the medical and scientific community, industry and international organizations, and regulators to help accomplish this task. Not many are fully aware of the amount of time that my fellow officers and I put in behind the scenes to expedite the medical products that could be used in the treatment of Ebola in the United States and abroad. Even though we were not in West Africa, we played a vital role. The FDA Ebola Response Team was crucial to the success of the FDA's response by issuing eleven emergency use authorizations, numerous emergency investigational new drug authorizations, and three international agreements of information sharing. Their unfailing leadership and work ethic exceeded the commitment that they were already required to do as part of their daily responsibilities and exemplified the extraordinary dedication to the FDA mission and the public health of this nation.

CDR Jamie Seligman

"Ebola is a caregiver's disease—the people who are at the greatest risk for infection are the caregivers."

—Jamie Seligman, LCSW-C, BCD

CDR Jamie Seligman served on the USPHS Commissioned Corps Ebola Response Mission at the Monrovia Medical Unit (MMU) in Margibi County, Liberia. He says, "As the lead of the behavioral health component, I supervised three psychologists, one psychiatrist, and one social worker. Our behavioral health team provided force health protection, spiritual care, and direct patient and family care. We collaborated with stakeholders such as the Liberian international healthcare workers operations, the Ministry of Health (MOH) and Social Welfare and the Carter Center staff. In our force health protection role[6], we conducted daily checks with officers who experienced challenges with the intensity of the work and high operation tempo, interpersonal relationship difficulties with colleagues, sleep hygiene problems, and coping with issues back home. Our behavioral health team provided strategies and interventions that ensured the best possible care for our patients and self-care for each officer. In addition, the behavioral health component cross-trained in donning, doffing, chlorine mixing, and other collateral duties as needed." In addition, the Substance Abuse and Mental Health Services Association (SAMHSA) Region 5 Administrator CAPT Jeff Coady, PsyD, played a vital role as the lead of the Behavioral Health Operations Group for the entire mission, coordinating behavioral health activities for officers during pre-deployment process, training, operations, and through reintegration. The Behavioral Health Operations Group was instrumental and ensured that vital information was flowing from Washington, DC, to Liberia, and vice versa. In addition, the team piloted the "Anticipate, Plan, and Deter" (APD) Responder Resilience System. For the Ebola response teams, APD included a pre-deployment responder stress inoculation training customized for this deployment. During this training, each responder developed an APD personal resilience plan that incorporated the training concepts for a personal strategy, taking into account anticipated stressors and individual coping and resilience resources. Officers were also trained in the Psychological Simple Triage and Rapid Treatment (PsySTART) Responder Self-Triage System, a rapid mental health triage tool for disaster or humanitarian missions.

CDR Seligman states, "PsySTART Responder allowed our officers to triage themselves daily. This empowered the officers to track the presence of their own risk markers and resilience, daily and cumulatively, across the extended course of the deployment. Over a period of days or weeks of deployment, officers tracked their own trends of risk factors over time. Armed with this information, the officers could elect to employ their personal resilience plans, developed during our initial training session in Anniston, Alabama, or they could share their daily triage or cumulative triage with the embedded behavioral health providers for additional coping ideas or support."

Officers were empowered to be proactive and or seek support resources in a timely manner. The self-triage information was aggregated automatically using the PsySTART responder system after personal information was removed. This approach to information helped to mitigate risk factors early, at both the individual and total team levels, rather than waiting for risk to become distress and disorder. CDR Seligman recalls, "For the past eight years, I have worked on disaster grants and have been deployed for disaster response many times. To be honest, my family would have been surprised if I had not been deployed. They are proud of the work that I do on a daily basis, and even

6—Force health protection is: "All services performed, provided, or arranged by the Services to promote, improve, conserve, or restore the mental or physical well-being of personnel." https://www.militaryfactory.com/dictionary/military-terms-defined.asp?term_id=2160

more proud of my work on the Ebola response when I can make a difference during such deployments." While there, CDR Seligman learned that "Ebola is a caregiver's disease—the people who are at the greatest risk for infection are the caregivers. It's a brother, sister, uncle, aunt, mother, father, or medical staff member who is taking care of the persons who are at the greatest risk of contracting the disease. Ebola affects the whole community and not just the individual."

To read the original (extended version) of this story, please visit: https://www.samhsa.gov/sites/default/files/dtac/dialogue-vol-12-issue-1.pdf

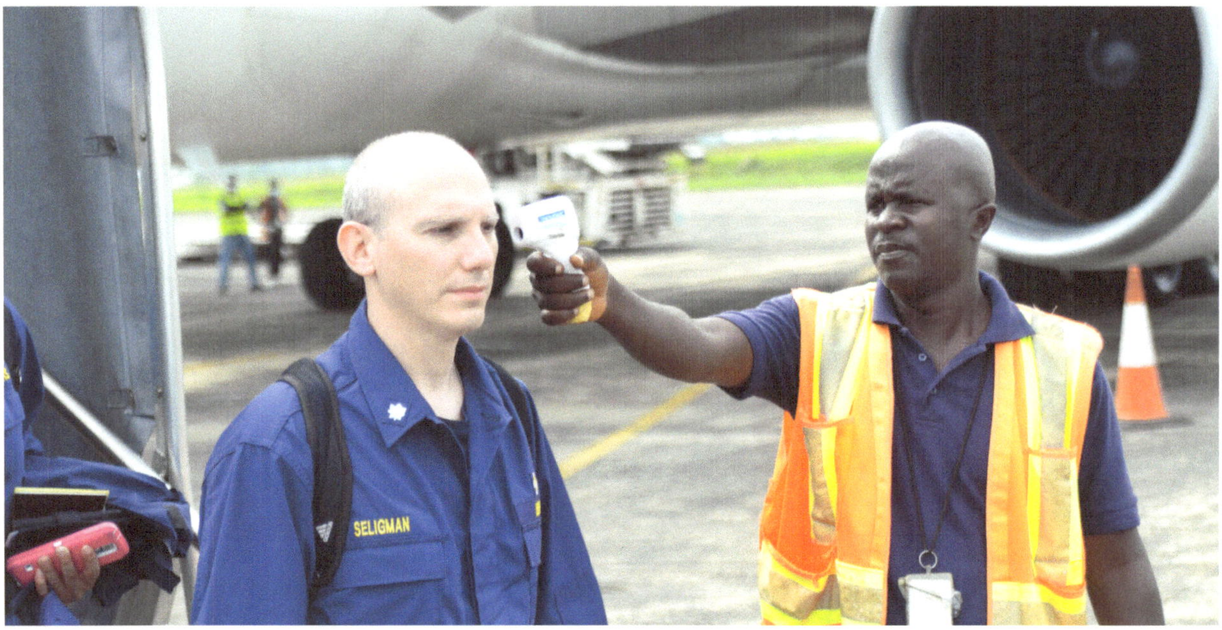

CDR Seligman's temperature is taken as he deplanes on the runway in Liberia.

CDR David Lau

"We brought hope in a crisis situation."

—David Lau, DPM

CDR David Lau was assigned to serve as the executive officer supporting RADM Trent-Adams and the Commissioned Corps Ebola Response mission to Liberia in any and all ways possible to ensure a successful outcome. CDR Lau speaks of getting the call to deploy: "It was Saturday, and I received a phone call. It was the United States Deputy Surgeon General (Acting) RADM Scott Giberson. It started off something like this: 'Hi CDR Lau. David. How are you doing? I need you to deploy to Liberia over the next two months. You have some key skill sets and experience we really need in Liberia!' 'Yes, Sir!' was my response to all questions. I proudly wore the USPHS Commissioend Corps uniform, and knew 'NO' was not an option! I made initial and final preparations at the same time, went down to San Diego to get my deployment physical, vaccinations, labs (thank you Navy Medicine for being so accommodating), and then shipped out to DC for some final preparations and State Department briefings before departing for Liberia! Kudos to our USPHS team for their above-and-beyond assistance in getting everything together for me! I was also advised to prepare a will. This was the REAL DEAL!!!"

Of his time in country, CDR Lau recalls, "In Liberia, I spent most of my time with RADM Trent-Adams, both at the Monrovia Medical Unit (MMU) and the United States Embassy, with duties that included assisting with and supporting the continuous operations of the MMU and United States government operations. I worked closely with the Disaster Assistance Response Team (DART) and the United States Army's 101st Airborne Division in ensuring the MMU received the necessary support and supplies to maintain operations. I also served as a representative of the United States response in communications and meetings with the Ministry of Health (MOH)

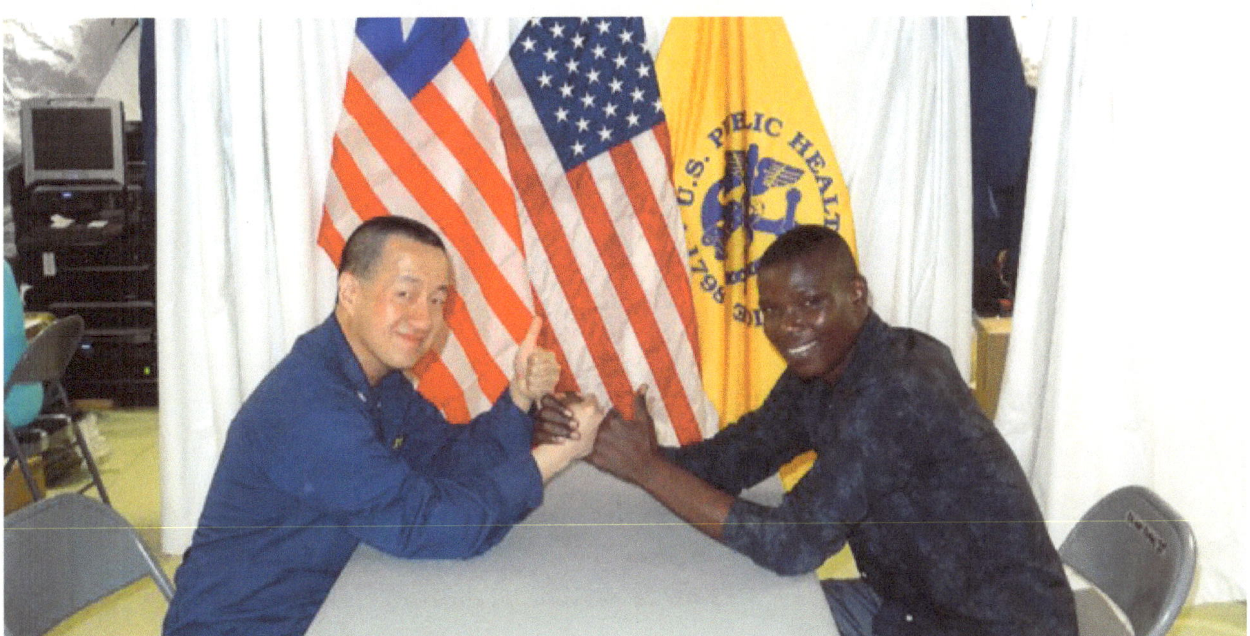

CDR Lau sits across the table from Liberian Physician Assistant Alvin Davis, the MMU's first Ebola survivor.

of Liberia, the United States, international VIPs, response teams, key stakeholders, and press. My daily routine involved preparations for the day, an 0700 working breakfast meeting, then meetings at the United States Embassy, off to the MMU (a forty-five minute drive), MMU work, and returning to the United States Embassy for a 1700 daily debriefing with United States leadership, followed by reporting, dinner, and closing out items for the day."

One of CDR Lau's first assignments was being the initial point of contact regarding Liberian and international healthcare workers referred to MMU for treatment. CDR Lau remembers, "I was given the hot phone! WOW! It could not get any more real than this!! We officially opened the MMU and received our first patient on November 12, 2014. He was a Liberian physician assistant. I also participated in the discussions and development of the Liberia Ebola Virus Disease (EVD) Clinical Management Manual with the World Health Organization (WHO) and the Liberian MOH. A critical assignment was to procure/secure critical medical equipment/supplies needed by the MMU from the leadership level."

Looking back now, CDR Lau shares, "This deployment was a defining moment and highlight in my career as a United States public health officer! I am very proud of the opportunity to serve and support our USPHS mission from a leadership perspective. We brought hope in a crisis situation. The entire world's eyes were on us. Once our USPHS Ebola hospital opened and started accepting healthcare patients, there was a genuine feeling of hope. As we accepted our first patients, and with the first discharges, everyone felt hope! And the world arrived and responded with numerous countries opening up additional Ebola Treatment Units (ETUs). We had led war against Ebola and won! I was honored to shake the hands of the first seven patients discharged from our hospital Ebola-free."

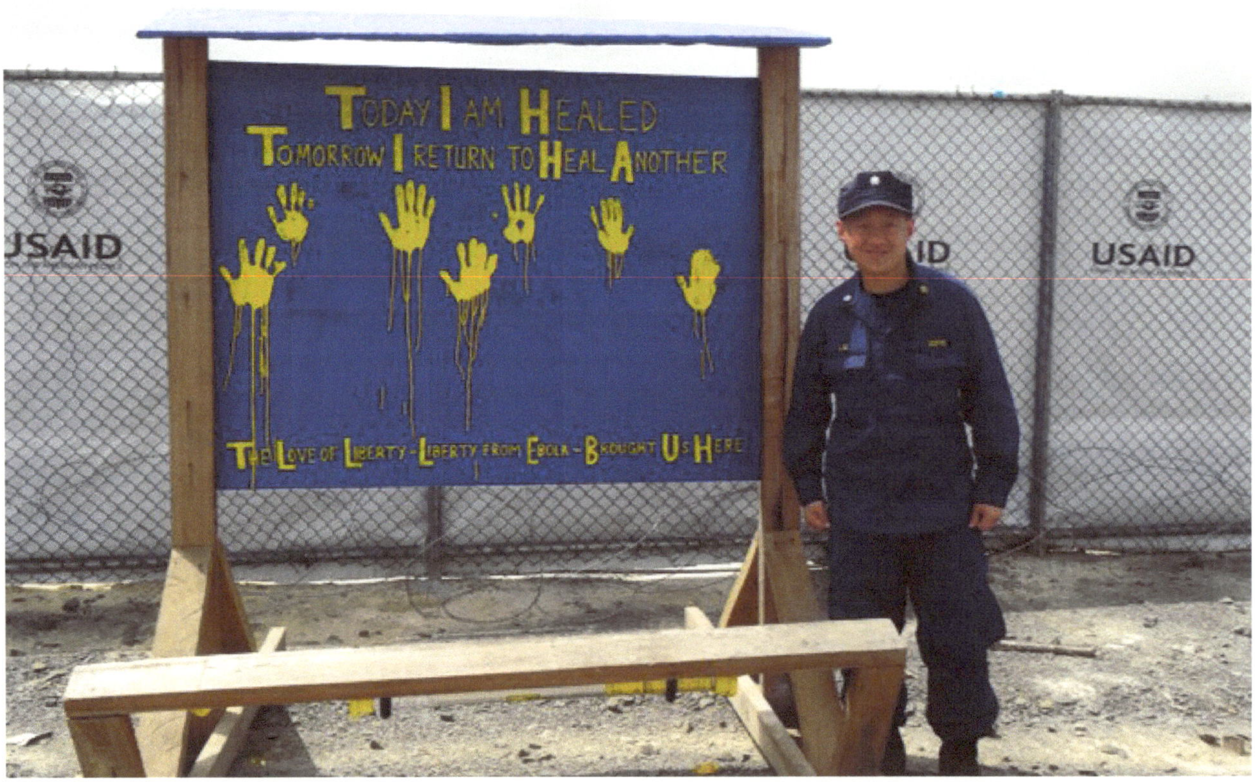
TODAY I AM HEALED
TOMORROW I RETURN TO HEAL ANOTHER
THE LOVE OF LIBERTY - LIBERTY FROM EBOLA - BROUGHT US HERE
USAID

CDR Lau stands to the right of the Ebola Survivor Wall. CDR Lau saw the first seven Ebola patients discharged.

CDR Tracy Pace

"... one of the most difficult adjustments that I had to make was 'distancing' myself from locals in order to protect myself."

—Tracy Pace, LCSW, MPH

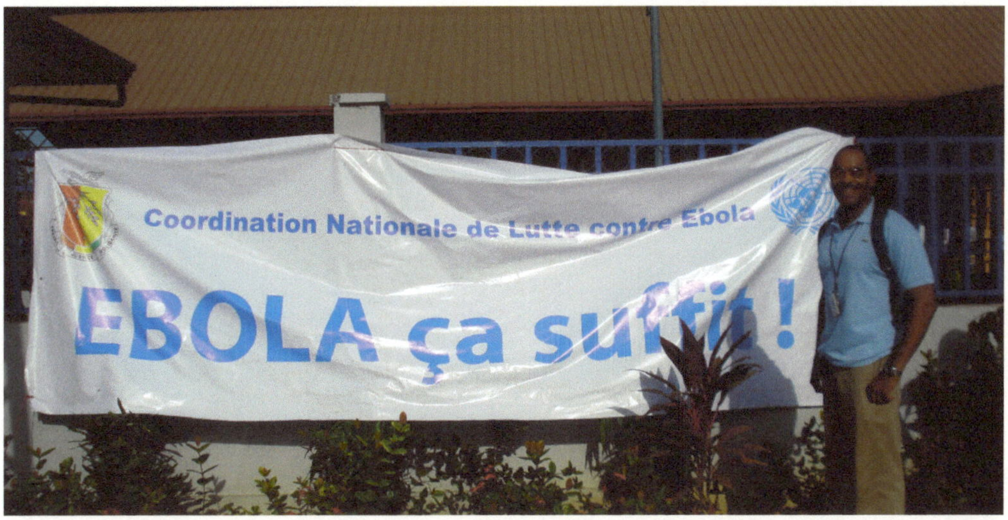

CDR Pace attends the launch of a major media campaign. In English, the sign read, "Ebola, that's enough!"

CDR Tracy Pace, with the Health Resources and Services Administration (HRSA), was one of about eleven French-speaking officers who were detailed to the Centers for Disease Control and Prevention (CDC) and subsequently deployed to Guinea, West Africa, for the Ebola response. Having had prior health education experience in West Africa, he was assigned to the Health Communication/Health Promotion Team for a deployment that lasted approximately forty-five days. The CDC–Guinea Health Communications Team, approximately five members strong, immediately began assessing what had been done to date and met with many international partners, including the United Nations Children's Fund, the World Health Organization, (WHO), Guinean media organizations, and various government ministry officials to determine what the current needs were. CDR Pace was responsible for monitoring the progress of health education and health communication activities undertaken by local non-governmental organizations (NGOs) that received CDC Foundation funding. Specifically, he met with NGO personnel to design realistic budgets, conducted site visits to observe activities and messaging, reviewed activity reports, recommended funding, and made payments. CDR Pace recalls, "Aside from having to come to terms with the extremely poor telecommunications infrastructure, one of the most difficult adjustments that I had to make was 'distancing' myself from locals in order to protect myself. I was a Peace Corps volunteer in Benin many years ago and was used to living, working, eating, and socializing with locals in my small Beninese village for almost two and a half years. I knew from the start of this Ebola response deployment that my experience in West Africa this time around wasn't going to be so convivial. It was hard to put limits on my interactions, but it was necessary in order that I not end up being 'that guy' that would have to be medevaced out of the country early and then showcased on the evening news in the United States due to my carelessness."

LCDR Jennifer Bornermann

"Christmas—and my life in general—will never be the same."

—Jennifer Bornermann, LCSW-C

LCDR Jennifer Bornermann was deployed as a behavioral health officer on Monrovia Medical Unit (MMU) Team 2, serving in Liberia from December 2014 to February 2015. She describes the work as challenging and heart-breaking, but also full of many highlights. LCDR Bornermann shares one story in which a group of officers had the distinct privilege of spending part of Christmas Day at an orphanage in Dolo Town, where children had lost one or both of their parents to Ebola: "We played games and sang with the children and also presented them with small gifts that our loved ones from home had sent us. (Thanks to the night shift, each gift was wrapped!)" On this day, LCDR Bornermann met Emmanuel. Emmanuel was a playfully shy nine-year-old boy who seemed to be enjoying the day with his friends. He would wink with a big smile as his way of saying "hi" and engaging with others. "When it was time for us to head back to the MMU, Emmanuel walked us back to the bus, which had gotten stuck in the mud a quarter-mile or so from the orphanage. I gave him a hug and wished him a good, productive life. As we drove away, one of my fellow officers pointed out the window to show me that Emmanuel continued running alongside the bus, waving to me. He ended up running about a mile until he could no longer keep up with us. Not a day goes by that I do not think about Emmanuel and wonder how he is doing. That sweet boy with a wink and smile left an imprint on my soul. Christmas—and my life in general—will never be the same."

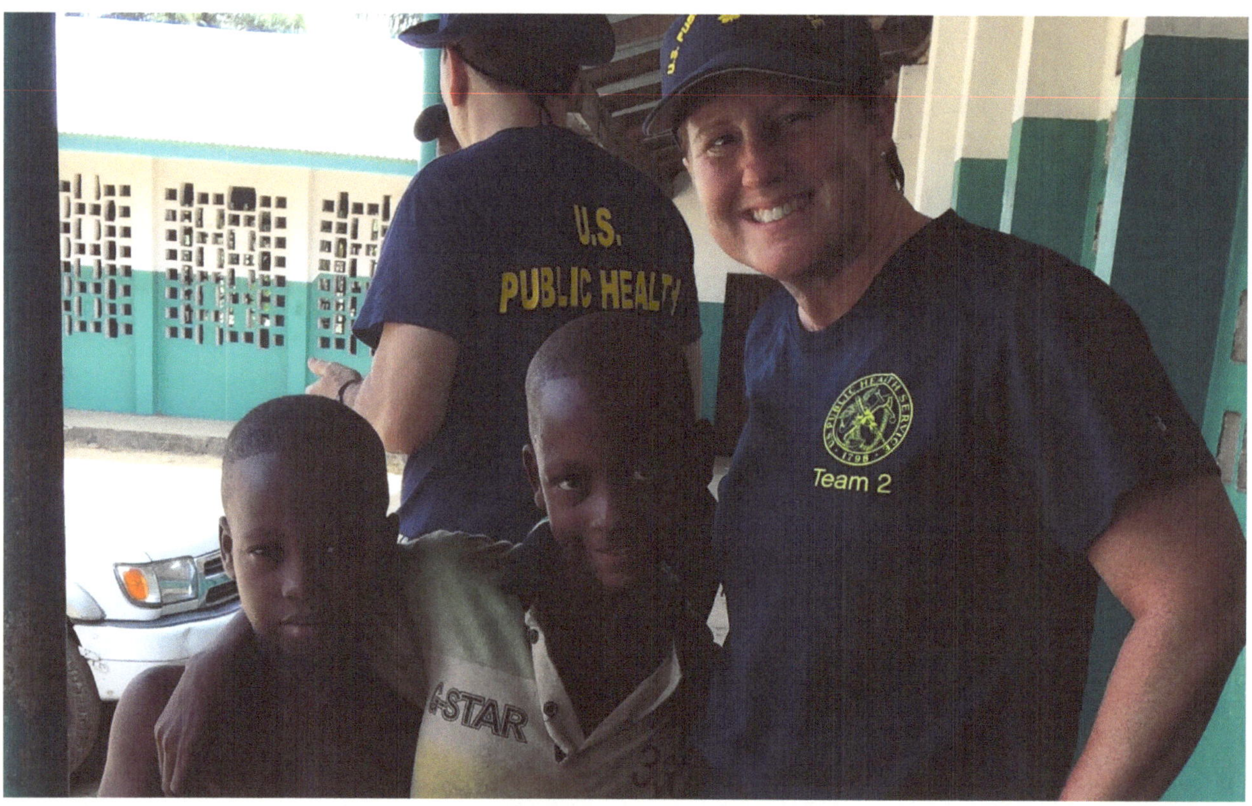

LCDR Bornermann *(right)* and Emmanuel to her immediate left, along with other little ones at the orphanage Christmas party.

LCDR Kate Migliaccio

"As families in Liberia cope with the fear, there are four words that offer a bit of comfort: 'The world is here.'"

—Kate Migliaccio, MPH

LCDR Kate Migliaccio served as the senior public information officer during the Ebola response. She recounts, "Our mission in West Africa is to care for the healthcare workers, so they, in turn, can care for the people in the region who have the disease. Shortly after I arrived in Liberia, I struck up a conversation with a Liberian security guard at the Monrovia Medical Unit (MMU). He told me about his dream of someday becoming a police officer in Monrovia. He also told me of a fear that had been wearing on him and his neighbors. 'Am I going to get Ebola?' he asked me. In a sense, that is the question the entire world had been asking. It is a question each of us asked ourselves at one point or another, ever since we learned of our mission. It is a question that has haunted many Americans as they watch the nightly news. And it most certainly is a very real question on the mind of just about every person who lives in West Africa. As families in Liberia cope with the fear, there are four words that offer a bit of comfort: 'The world is here.' We are in West Africa to offer help, healing, and hope—continuing the legacy of our Corps and our country. When our neighbors need us most, we Americans open our hearts and extend our hands—regardless of whether they live in places near or far. In this sense we are there to be hope multipliers. To offer those 'ripples of hope' Robert Kennedy talked about years ago. Ripples that together form a current that alters the course of this deadly outbreak. To alter the course, that is, to save lives, we need safe facilities and safe equipment, and most importantly, we need to keep the people safe who are doing the saving. I keep thinking about that security guard, and what our being

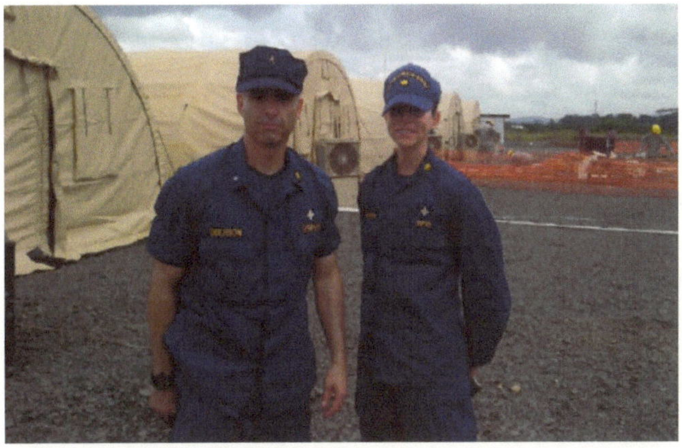

LCDR Migliaccio *(right)* stands alongside RADM Giberson (acting US Deputy Surgeon General) at the MMU.

there means to him, his family, and his future. While he didn't have the disease itself, he had been living with the fear and worry that came with it, so it meant so much to him to finally have some hope, and to know we are there to care for healthcare workers. He said that our help in containing this outbreak means that people like him can go back to living their daily lives with a sense of a safer and more secure future. It also means that he can now pursue his dream of becoming a police officer. He couldn't stop thanking me, and he asked me to thank the American people when I got back home. For those of us here in the United States, our work means that we, too, can have a greater sense of safety and security. That's why I'm so proud of the . . . incredible Commissioned Corps officers who've left their homes and families to volunteer for the MMU mission.[7]"

7—Originally published November 17, 2014, at https://wayback.archive-it.org/8315/20170119054514/https:/www.hhs.gov/blog/2014/11/17/offering-help-healing-and-hope-liberia.html

LCDR Chris Poulson

"It was very exciting and rewarding to see patients survive Ebola, be discharged, and be reunited with their families."

—Chris Poulson, PsyD, LSOTP, ABPP

LCDR Poulson was deployed with Monrovia Medical Unit (MMU) Team 1 as a psychologist. He recalls, "At that time, there was a palpable anxiety related to fears that Ebola Virus Disease (EVD) was spreading like wildfire across West Africa and the same might happen here in the states. When I deployed, a second case of EVD was confirmed here in Dallas, hitting very close to home." For the deployment, LCDR Poulson's primary role was force health protection, providing psychological services to USPHS Commissioned Corps officers. He shares, "We prepared at the Center for Domestic Preparedness (CDP) in Anniston, Alabama. We learned what was known about EVD. I was able to 'inoculate' MMU Team 1 members with a personalized protection plan designed to assist officers in managing the stress of working in the Ebola Treatment Unit (ETU). We practiced how to safely work in a mock ETU contaminated with GloGerm while wearing personal protective equipment (PPE). The experience was sobering." In addition, LCDR Poulson provided limited psychological services to patients infected with EVD. Of course, USPHS Commissioned Corps officers take on other duties as assigned. Therefore, he assisted with doffing, cleaning beds in the hot zone of the ETU, and removing biohazardous waste from the hot zone to the incinerators. Of this deployment, LCDR Poulson says, "It was very exciting and rewarding to see patients survive Ebola, be discharged, and be reunited with their families. Facing formidable foes during the mission, I forged lifelong friendships. It was gratifying to be ready and willing to successfully serve our country at what felt like a pivotal time in history."

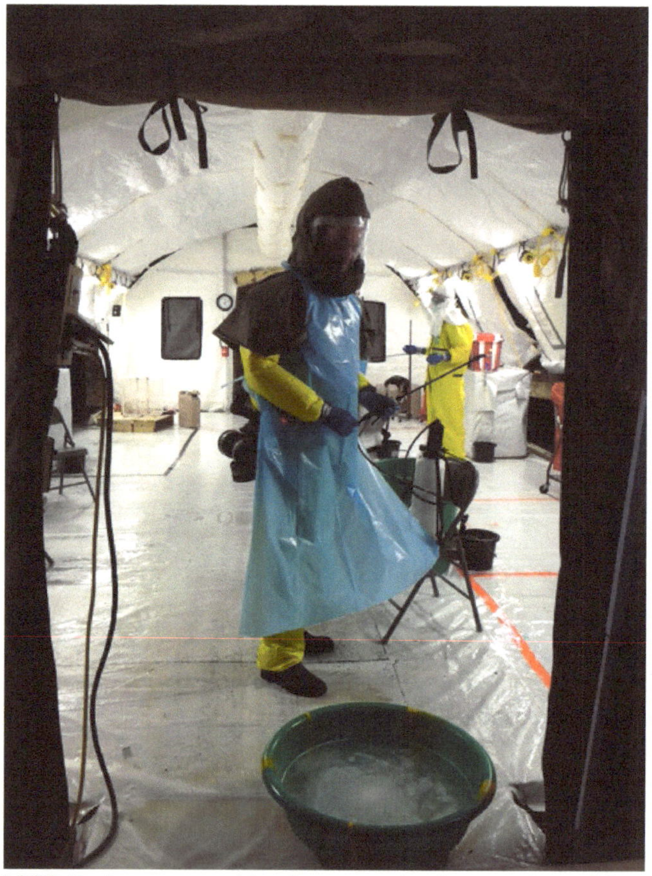

LCDR Poulson uses a bleach sprayer to decontaminate fellow officers in Liberia during the doffing process.

LCDR Skip Payne

"I was able to experience and communicate firsthand the positive impact that effective federal, state, and local partnerships can have during a public health emergency. . ."

—Skip Payne, MSPH, REHS/RS, CPH, CHEP

LCDR Skip Payne served as a Health and Human Services (HHS) subject matter expert on national volunteer programs and related issues for the HHS Secretary's Operation Center (SOC) Emergency Management Group's Ebola Virus Disease (EVD) Taskforce. He also served as a Medical Reserve Corps (MRC) program liaison to the HHS SOC. The information and situational awareness he provided to the SOC informed decision-making at the federal level, better enabling HHS and federal partners to complement and support state and local HHS departments' preparedness and response activities. He recalls, "I struggled with the fact that I was not able to deploy to Liberia but was happy to be called upon to serve in this way." LCDR Payne was originally slated to deploy; however, due to an imminent program need that matched his unique skillset, he was deemed mission critical by his program leadership and asked to stay in Washington, DC. As part of his role as the MRC program liaison to the HHS SOC, LCDR Payne was proud to represent the work of the state and local MRC units for this event. Two notable units were the Dallas County MRC in Dallas, Texas, and the MRC of Hennepin County in Hopkins, Minnesota.

LCDR Payne led a team that helped to ensure the SOC was aware of the work that these units were doing to ensure federal resources did not overlap with locally available services and that national-level standardized trainings were communicated to the MRC Network when they became available. The Dallas County MRC and MRC units surrounding the first domestic case of this outbreak supported a call center, serving a total of 579 hours over a nineteen-day period. Volunteers also dedicated time to hand out materials provided by the Centers for Disease Control and Prevention (CDC) and conducted neighborhood canvassing. The Dallas County MRC unit also provided training for the use of personal protective equipment (PPE) and a psychological first aid course that was offered to community providers, mental health and social work professionals, counselors, chaplains, and non-medical volunteers. Additionally, the MRC of Hennepin County (Hopkins, Minnesota) coordinated with partners from the local Cultural Services Unit (CSU) to hold its first regional training for all MRC CSU volunteers from the three jurisdictions the unit serves. The training focused on peer education, using Ebola as an example of a current public health emergency for which peer education can be used to disseminate information to the general public. The training included an orientation to peer education as a public health concept, a panel discussion of experts to talk about Ebola, and a small group exercise for participants to practice using peer education skills when asked questions about Ebola. After the training session, the MRC CSU deployed volunteers and the MRC coordinator to distribute Ebola health education materials and organize a community information session on Ebola. The MRC coordinator also shared a copy of the unit's CSU resources with the MRC Network as a tool for other leaders to use and replicate. LCDR Payne's experience during the Ebola response—including his specific role on the EVD taskforce and representing the work of state and local MRC units—was rewarding, challenging, and eye-opening. He recalls, "I was able to experience and communicate firsthand the positive impact that effective federal, state, and local partnerships can have during a public health emergency and witness the power of volunteers willing and able to help their communities during times of need."

LCDR Matthew Johns

"I often reflect on how truly humbling Ebola is as a disease in any setting and how challenging the clinical course was for all of our patients. They remain the true heroes in all of this."

—Matthew Johns, MPH

LCDR Matthew Johns served as the chief of preventive medicine with Monrovia Medical Unit (MMU) Team 2. He recounts that "as an infectious disease epidemiologist by training, the deployment was something that most people work their entire career to be part of. I still have vivid memories of how we would all gather around after donning our personal protective equipment (PPE), but before we would go into the hot zone. We would discuss the plan of action among the five- to seven-person team, we would all stand in a circle, take deep breaths, touch elbows, and collectively calm ourselves before entering. Every move was accounted for by preventive medicine safety staff. Every clinical step was carefully choreographed among the group. I often reflect on how truly humbling Ebola is as a disease in any setting and how challenging the clinical course was for all of our patients. They remain the true heroes in all of this. I will never forget them and never forget the officers whom I stood 'elbow-to-elbow' with in the fight. The unique clinical mission truly set the USPHS Commissioned Corps apart from the other United States government responders. It put us in a position to support multiple countries and fellow healthcare workers in the battle against this extremely deadly disease."

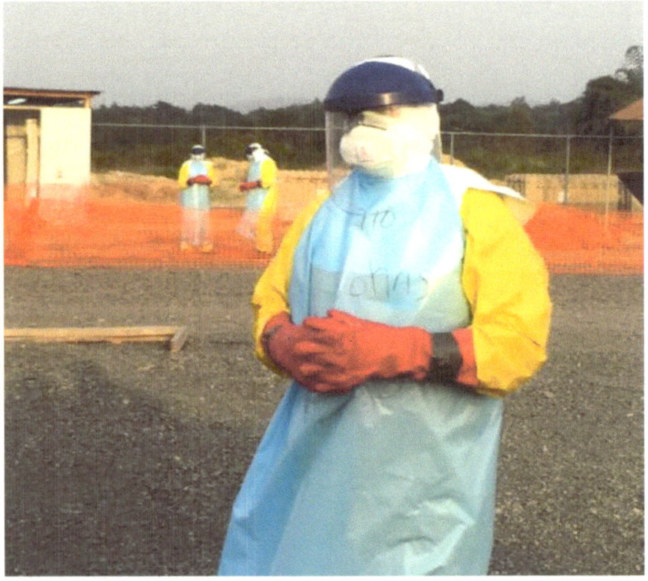

(front) LCDR Johns, MMU, Preventive Medicine Chief; *(back left)* CAPT de la Cruz, MMU Deputy Officer-in-Charge (DOIC); *(back right)* and CAPT Dickens, MMU Officer-in-Charge (OIC), prepare to transport highly-infectious biowaste within the hot zone.

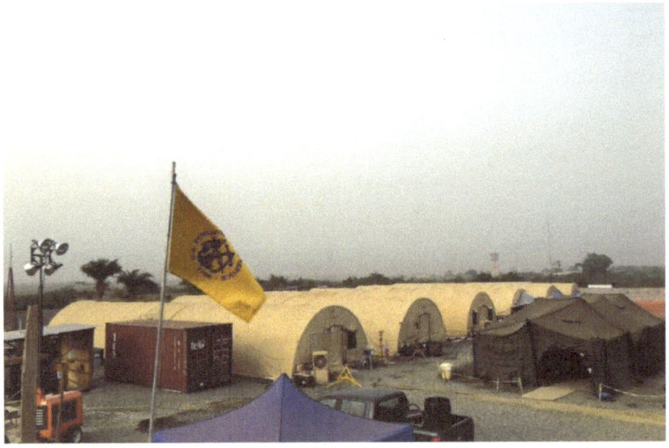

The USPHS flag flying high atop the MMU.

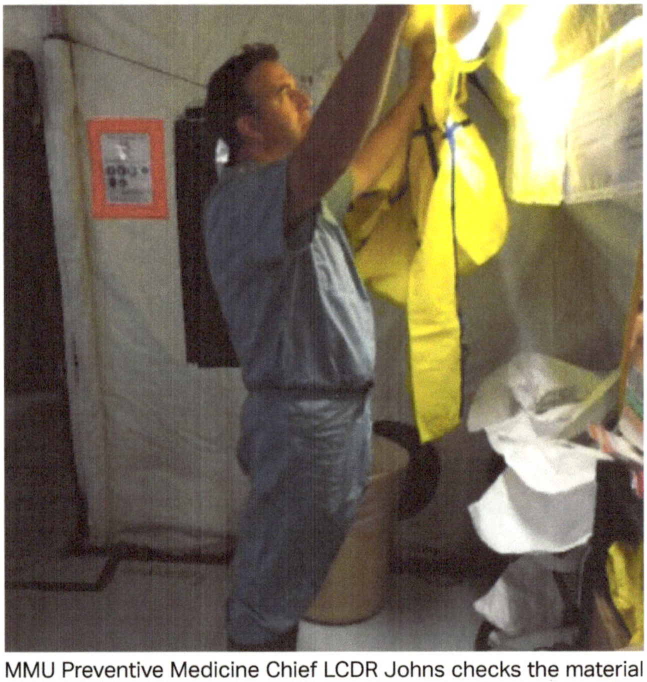

MMU Preventive Medicine Chief LCDR Johns checks the material of his PPE for holes and small flaws prior to donning and entering the hot zone.

LCDR Philip Lafleur

"The friends and memories made will last our lifetimes, as will the impact of our work here."

—Philip Lafleur, MPA, PAC

LCDR Philip Lafleur deployed to Monrovia, Liberia, from October 17 until December 23, 2014, as a Force Health physician's assistant at the Monrovia Medical Unit (MMU). LCDR Lafleur shares that his reflections regarding this deployment are now very different than they were at the beginning. "When we arrived in Liberia we were filled with excitement and idealistic hopes. We were so glad to have been privileged enough to be chosen for this historic, high-profile mission. There was so much work to get ready both training in Anniston, Alabama, before we left and setting up an Ebola treatment facility in a mobile Air Force hospital once we arrived. There were tons of high-profile visitors and journalists that provided publicity both in the United States and worldwide. That early time was a rush, a blur of days and events. Then came the momentous day we received our first patient, a very sick man who we are virtually positive would have not survived without our intervention. He was followed by many others. Some survived and some did not. We did our best with the training, experience, and equipment we had to work with."

LCDR Lafleur recalls that his role was as the force health physician assistant, but since the majority of the staff were medical professionals, many with prescriptive privileges, the majority of his time was not spent on force health protection. "During our days in Liberia, I think I treated perhaps thirty team members. On two occasions, my role came to the forefront. Once, when we first arrived and several members of the team got traveler's diarrhea from drinking the local water, although nearly every one of them had brought a small pharmacy for such contingencies, and they self-medicated successfully. The other was in the doffing tent when choline fumes were causing team members to choke and cough as they entered the hot zone. Ultimately we rolled the flaps up to air the tent out and that solved the problem." Because the force health role was not all-consuming, LCDR Lafleur also served as the day shift hall monitor. "Once someone enters the hot zone they cannot come out; it is a one-way path to keep the virus contained. So if they needed anything, someone had to be available to get it. That person needed a modicum of medical training because it might be a device or medication that was needed."

Of the deployment, LCDR Lafleur recounts that "a lot of effort went into enduring the long hours and difficult circumstances. We rejoiced in what benefits we did have, like hot showers and air conditioning, and endured others, like the long, dusty bus ride to and from the treatment center each day and weeks of eating MREs. Now I think about what could have been done better, what might have been if circumstances had been different? No deployment every works out well 100 percent. I'm very pleased with our successes and deeply disappointed by our inabilities to succeed in some instances." He expresses that "throughout our time in Liberia, in the midst of concentrating on our mission, our thoughts were constantly of what we'd do when we get home and how much we miss our families, our country and our 'lives.' I am very content to have done this; to have been here with these fine men and women and to have taken on an insidious enemy for the protection, promotion, and advancement of the public health of the Liberian people, and ultimately the people of the whole earth. The friends and memories made will last our lifetimes as will the impact of our work here. Though it has been nearly four years, this is heady stuff, and it humbles me still."

LCDR Karen Forbes

"It was rewarding to be able to contribute to this historic response."

—Karen Forbes, MPA-S, PA-C

LCDR Karen Forbes served as the physician assistant and lead deployment coordinator for the Centers for Disease Control and Prevention (CDC) Occupational Health Clinic (OHC). She was involved in the Ebola response for the entire duration of the response. She worked on the pre-and post-deployment efforts of the agency. Through the OHC, she coordinated medical clearances for over 3,400 CDC and other Health and Human Services (HHS) staff detailed as part of the agency's response effort. Along with the CDC OHC medical team, she was involved in completing medical clearances to ensure those being sent out were medically suited for emergency response to the Ebola outbreak. During the first six months of the Ebola response, LCDR Forbes conducted 268 Ebola post-deployment assessments of returning CDC and other HHS staff. She also conducted weekly monitoring during the twenty-one days post-deployment for symptoms of Ebola for the first six months of the response. During this time, she consulted with Ebola subject matter experts on a regular basis. This effort ensured that staff returned safely to their posts and protected the workplace and public, both stateside and internationally. LCDR Forbes states, "It was rewarding to be able to contribute to this historic response."

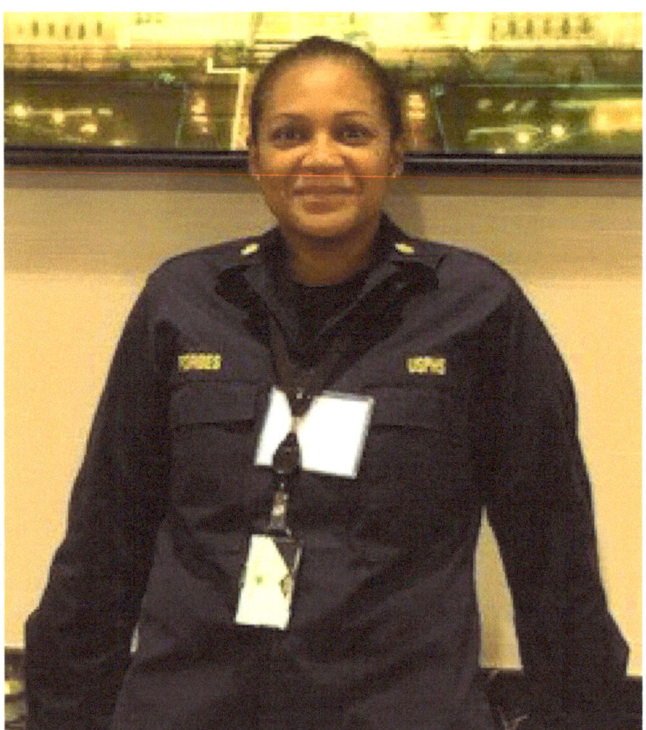

LCDR Forbes pauses for a quick photo despite a hectic support schedule.

LCDR Rafael Torres-Cruz

"It was a great responsibility to ensure the welfare of the patients and the safety and security of fellow officers, especially ensuring their safe return home to their loved ones."

—Rafael Torres-Cruz MS, MPH, ADC

LCDR Rafael Torres-Cruz served on Monrovia Medical Unit (MMU) Team 1. Following the news of the situation in Liberia, there were rumors about the possibility of a USPHS Commissioned Corps deployment to Liberia. Days later, LCDR Torres-Cruz was contacted by CDR DeGrange to participate in the initial response. He immediately agreed to join the team going to Liberia. LCDR Torres-Cruz knew the stakes were high because he was part of the safety team and was the only officer with experience working with biological agents in high and maximum containment. He shares, "It was a great responsibility to ensure the welfare of the patients and the safety and security of fellow officers, especially ensuring their safe return home to their loved ones." That was his goal towards all the officers when working in the hot zone. LCDR Torres-Cruz was assigned to the night shift to ensure the safety of his fellow officers. He escorted officers to the hot zone every single time a team member entered the zone. As a result, he entered the hot zone at least three times every single night. He finally took a day of rest after twenty-eight consecutive nights. He did not return to a normal routine until the last day of deployment, when his team properly trained MMU Team 2 and turned over the command of the MMU. He states that "MMU Team 1 was such a unique team. Everyone was so dedicated and supportive. The leadership was incredible, and the team became a big family." Upon returning to the states, CAPT Edwards and LCDR Torres-Cruz were the last ones to return home; there was no transition or acclimation, just the honor and reward of serving their country during a time of need.

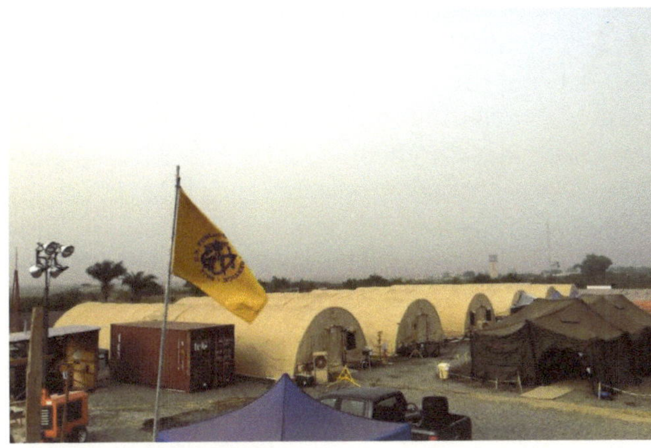

PHS flag flying over Camp Eason.

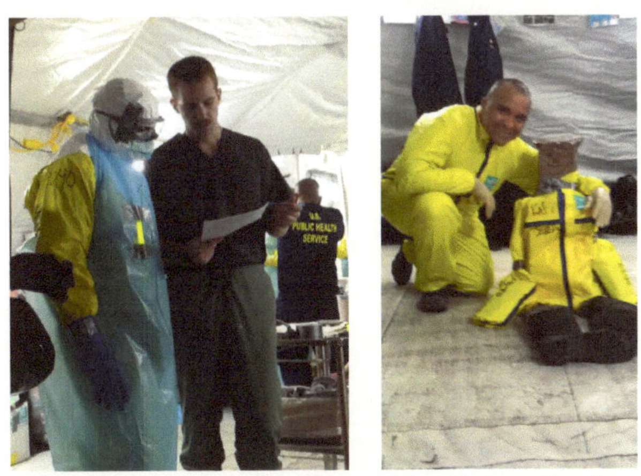

(left) LCDR Torres-Cruz receiving additional information from LT Simpson prior to entering the MMU hot zone. *(right)* Rafi 2, named after LCDR Torres-Cruz, was created by the night shift using MRE boxes and extra personal protective equipment (PPE). The mannequin was used to practice patient evacuation drills.

LCDR Julie Erb-Alvarez

"One of the most meaningful aspects of my deployment was the joy felt by our team when a patient was discharged from the Monrovia Medical Unit and was able to place their yellow hand print on the Survivor's Wall."

—Julie Erb-Alvarez, MPH, CPH

As a planning officer, one of LCDR Julie Erb-Alvarez's duties was managing communications for Monrovia Medical Unit (MMU) Team 2, including mobile communications and newsletter development. LCDR Erb-Alvarez purchased local mobile devices and SIM cards as requested by team members and leadership. This duty could be logistically challenging, but it was crucial and provided a morale boost for team members. LCDR Erb-Alvarez states, "The ability to communicate with our families at home was vital, especially over the holidays, as we were in the country over Christmas and New Year's." When mobile devices broke, which was often, or officers ran out of minutes, LCDR Erb-Alvarez worked with the local company to alleviate the problem. She also produced a daily newsletter for the team to boost morale and provide critical information on a regular basis.

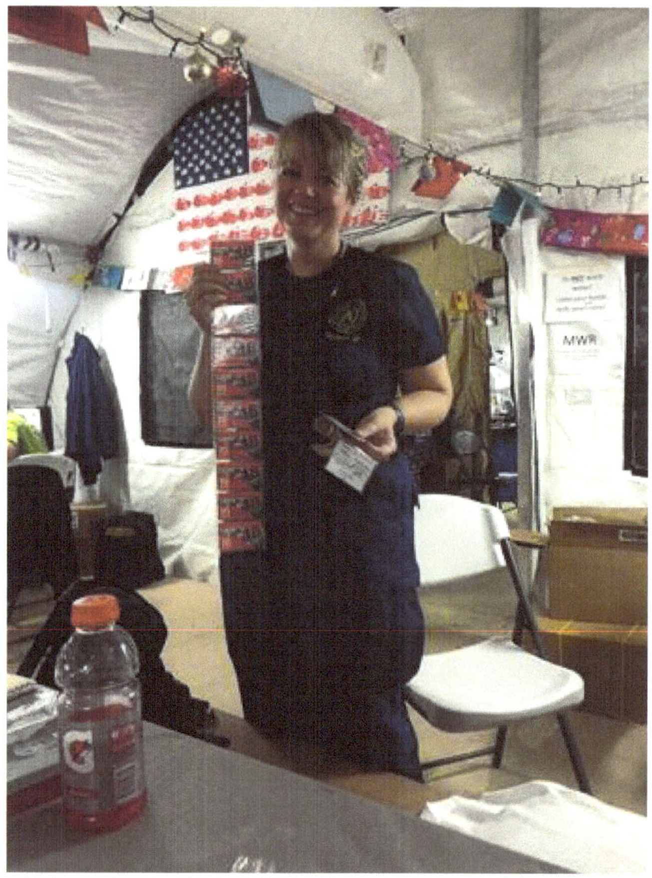

LCDR Erb-Alvarez at the MMU with Liberian phone airtime scratch cards.

Aside from this and other vital planning operations, LCDR Erb-Alvarez served as a doffer, assisting officers exiting the hot zone while guiding them through the twenty-six steps of removing personal protective equipment (PPE), where attention to detail can mean life or death. This was a critical and meticulous process for infection prevention. "I truly enjoyed my work at the MMU. I enjoyed writing each and every newsletter and now look back on them as historical documents detailing our time in West Africa. One of the most meaningful aspects of my deployment was the joy felt by our team when a patient was discharged from the Monrovia Medical Unit and was able to place their yellow hand print on the Survivor's Wall."

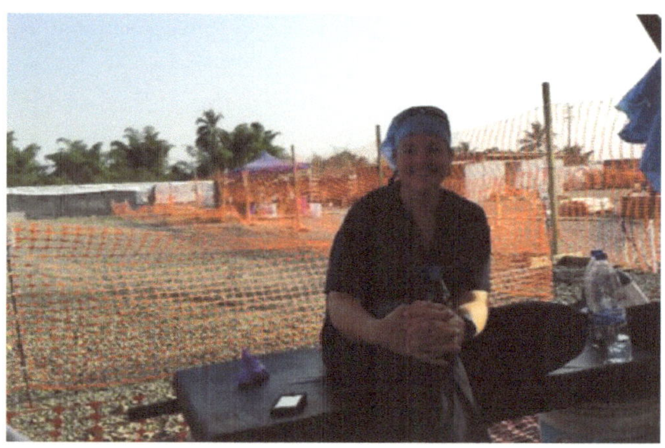

LCDR Erb-Alvarez sitting outside the hot zone waiting for the next officer to doff.

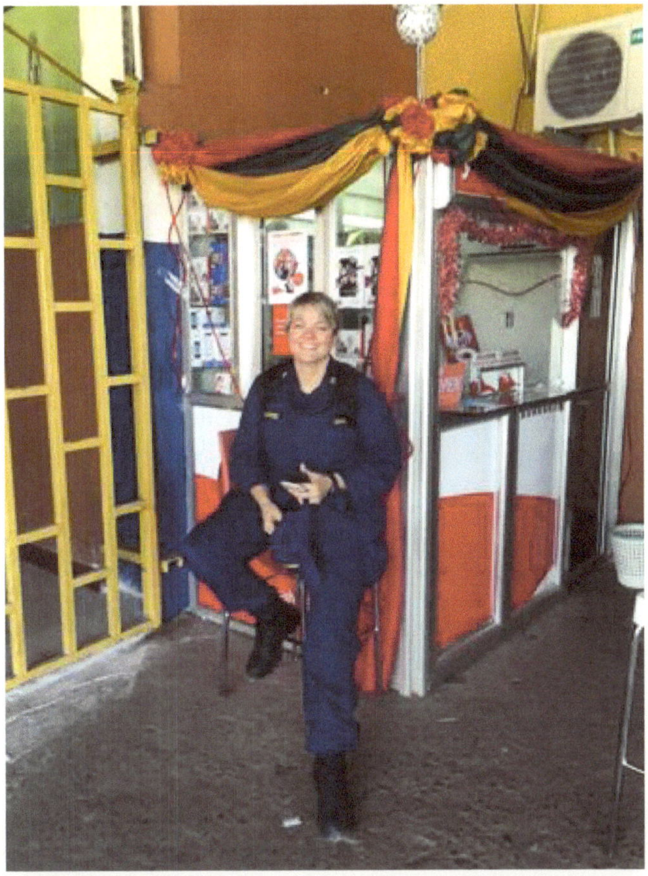

LCDR Erb-Alvarez at the phone store located at Roberts International Airport in Monrovia. The store was actually the booth shown behind her in this photo.

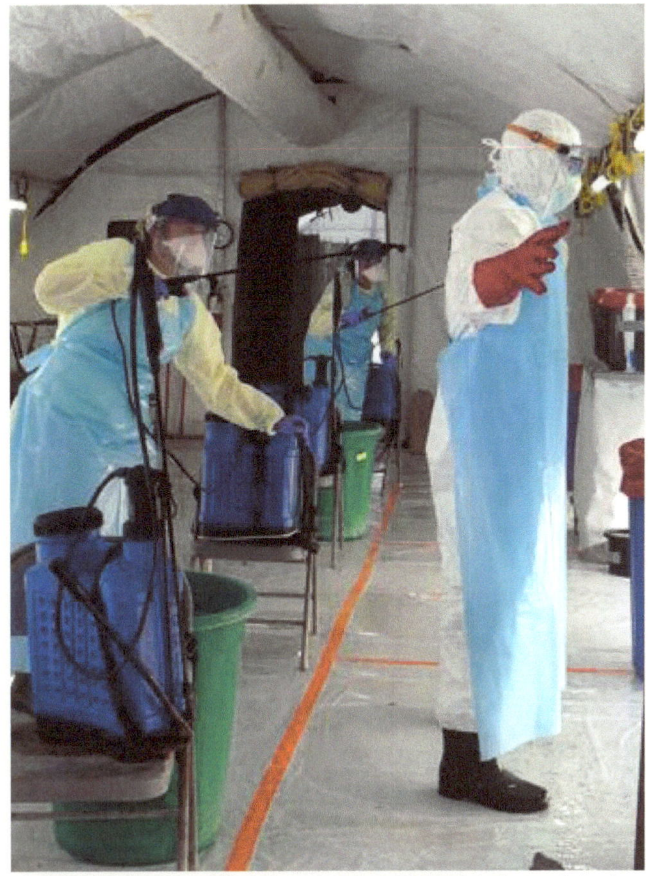

LCDR Erb-Alvarez doffing Laboratorian CDR Christl out of the hot zone.

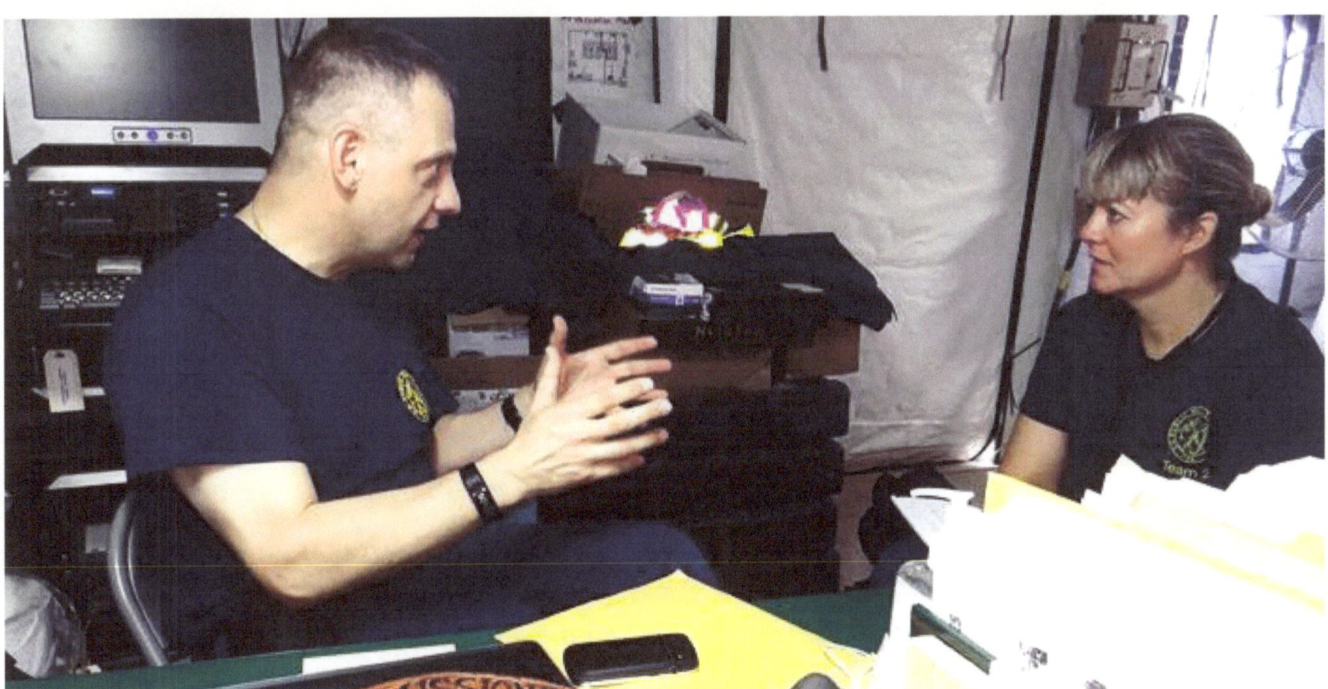

LCDR Erb-Alvarez interviews RADM Lushniak for the officer spotlight section of the MMU Team 2 newsletter.

LCDR Evelyn Seel

"It was a very inspiring activity to be able to support families emotionally while their loved ones were deployed."

—Evelyn Seel, MPH

LCDR Evelyn Seel was part of the United States Public Health Service (USPHS) Monrovia Medical Unit (MMU) Family Support Network (FSN). The role of an FSN volunteer included reaching out to a designated family and explaining the resources available to them, both physical and psychological. Volunteers were trained in communication techniques for phone and email. They were not intended to be counselors but rather supported and connected family members with information and resources while a loved one was deployed.

LCDR Seel supported two families during the MMU Team 1 deployment. Her duties included answering questions; responding to concerns; and linking families to USPHS support resources, webinars, and conference calls. She also helped LT Tracy Tilghman draft the FSN standard operations procedures. LCDR Seel states, "It was a very inspiring activity to be able to support families emotionally while their loved ones were deployed. Several meaningful connections have endured."

LT Tracy Tilghman

"I think that the officers and their families appreciated the care and support, which made all the stress, sleepless nights, and organized craziness worth it."

—Tracy Tilghman, MPH, MSW, CHES

LT Tracy Tilghman developed and implemented the Family Support Network (FSN) to assist the families of officers deploying to the Monrovia Medical Unit (MMU) in Liberia. The first of its kind for USPHS Commissioned Corps officers, the FSN provided ongoing communication and transparency between mission activities, family members of deployed officers, and USPHS entities. The FSN also conducted training, educated volunteers and FSN staff on roles and responsibilities, and developed and implemented weekly information sessions for families of deployed officers.

On a personal level, the FSN was a way for LT Tilghman to help her fellow officers. "A lot of my team members deployed with MMU Team 1, so I had a vested interest in making sure their families had the support they needed, were able to communicate with their loved ones, and were kept abreast of what was occurring downrange. A lot of what occurred in that first month was thanks to my expertise, my background as an Air Force brat, and the experiences my family had with family support during that time. The rest was just intuition," says LT Tilghman. "I literally ate, drank, and breathed FSN, working twenty-four hours a day for close to two months to ensure continuity of operations and that everything ran smoothly. Sure, there were bumps along the way, but I and those couple officers who assisted in the very beginning worked hard to make things look seamless for officers and their families. In the end, I think that the officers and their families appreciated the care and support, which made all the stress, sleepless nights, and organized craziness worth it."

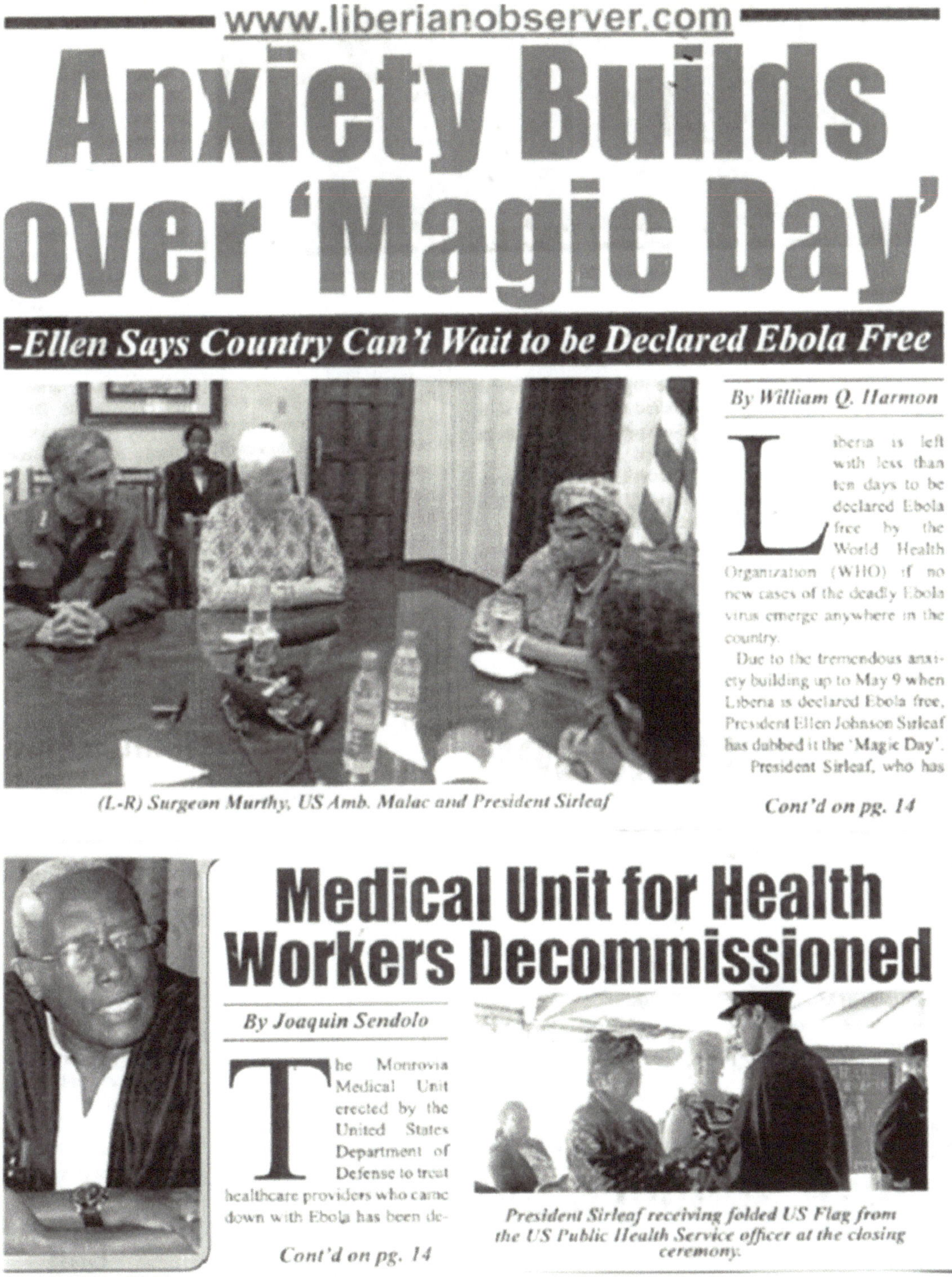

www.liberianobserver.com

Anxiety Builds over 'Magic Day'

-Ellen Says Country Can't Wait to be Declared Ebola Free

(L-R) Surgeon Murthy, US Amb. Malac and President Sirleaf

By William Q. Harmon

Liberia is left with less than ten days to be declared Ebola free by the World Health Organization (WHO) if no new cases of the deadly Ebola virus emerge anywhere in the country.

Due to the tremendous anxiety building up to May 9 when Liberia is declared Ebola free, President Ellen Johnson Sirleaf has dubbed it the 'Magic Day'.

President Sirleaf, who has

Cont'd on pg. 14

Medical Unit for Health Workers Decommissioned

By Joaquin Sendolo

The Monrovia Medical Unit erected by the United States Department of Defense to treat healthcare providers who came down with Ebola has been de-

Cont'd on pg. 14

President Sirleaf receiving folded US Flag from the US Public Health Service officer at the closing ceremony.

The above article, titled "Anxiety Builds over 'Magic Day'," was taken from the Liberian Observer on May 1, 2015. It shows Surgeon General Dr. Vivek Murthy presenting a folded US flag to Liberian President Ellen Johnson-Sirleaf in recognition of the US decommissioning of the Monrovia Medical Unit (MMU)[8].

8—https://www.liberianobserver.com/news/anxiety-builds-over-magic-day/

LCDR Lorraine Williams

"Coordinating with Walter Reed and local health departments was the most memorable part of my service . . ."

—Lorraine Williams, DHSc, MSc, CHES

LCDR Lorraine Williams was a part of the new reintegration specialist role that was established for the Ebola deployment. This involved serving officers that were deployed and helping them get reintegrated at home and at their duty stations. LCDR Williams' day-to-day role was to provide support to officers and monitoring daily temperatures. She prepared reports for federal and local health departments where the officer resided. Each reintegration specialist had different challenges. LCDR Williams says, "Coordinating with Walter Reed and local health departments was the most memorable part of my service because two of the officers assigned to me required medical care." LCDR Williams would love to serve in this role again.

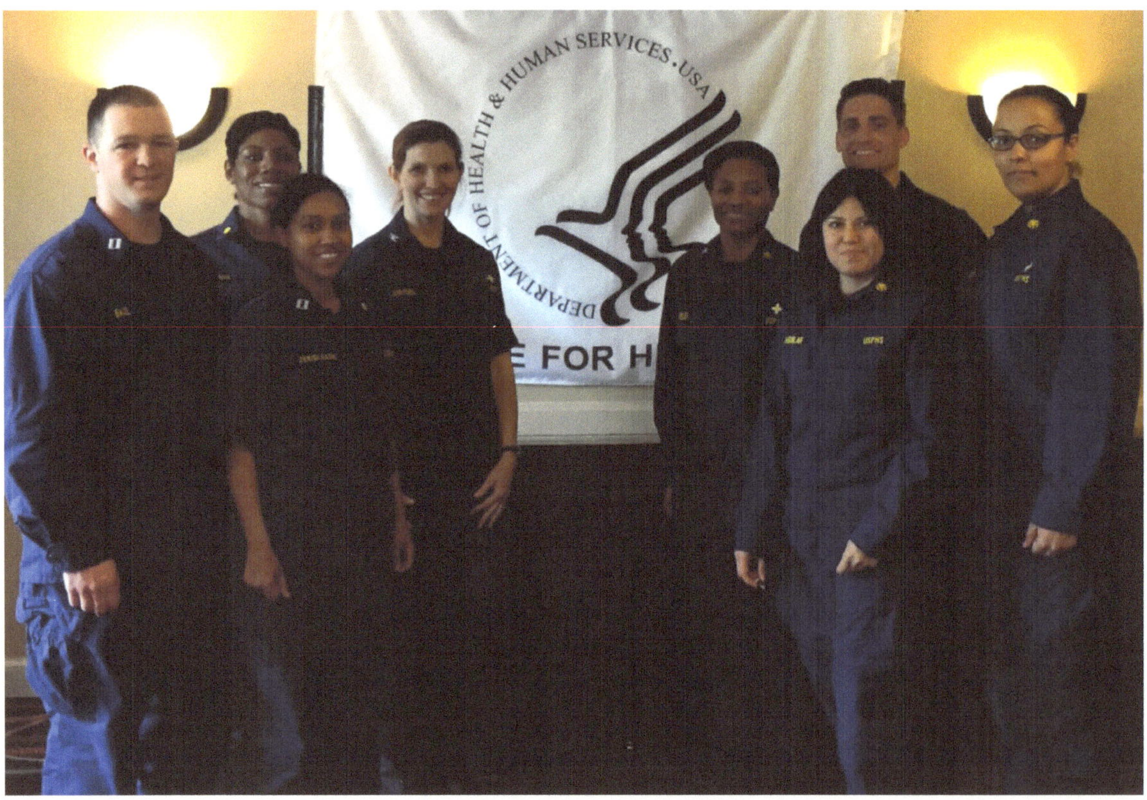

LCDR Williams *(back left)* poses with the MMU-4 Reintegration Team in front of the Department of Health and Human Services flag.

LT Jennifer Freiman

"While I am proud of my personal contributions to the response, I am most proud of our team, a group of officers who put service before self and worked together to accomplish the mission and ensure everyone returned home safely."

—Jennifer Freiman, MPH, CPH

LT Freiman deployed to Liberia with Monrovia Medical Unit (MMU) Team 4 in the planning section. Her primary responsibilities were to produce daily situational reports, facilitate internal team communication, create and maintain daily schedules, plan team activities, and prepare after-action reports. She also provided epidemiology support and served as a doffer. During the final week of her deployment, LT Freiman was detailed to Sierra Leone to support an Ebola vaccine trial with the Centers for Disease Control and Prevention (CDC). LT Freiman supported enrollment activities and conducted a process evaluation for one of the laboratory components of the trial.

Three years later, LT Freiman still thinks about the strong and resilient people she met in Liberia and Sierra Leone. Many of the nationals that she met were extremely appreciative and surprised that responders would leave their homes and families to help. She was proud to represent the USPHS Commissioned Corps and had the opportunity to meet responders from organizations and countries all over the world. LT Freiman witnessed firsthand the importance of partnerships and collaboration, and she returned home motivated to gain a better understanding of how to navigate the complexities and challenges of working in the global health arena. LT Freiman is currently pursuing a graduate certificate in global health engagement from the Uniformed Services University of the Health Sciences.

LT Freiman states, "While I am proud of my personal contributions to the response, I am most proud of our team, a group of officers who put service before self and worked together to accomplish the mission and ensure everyone returned home safely."

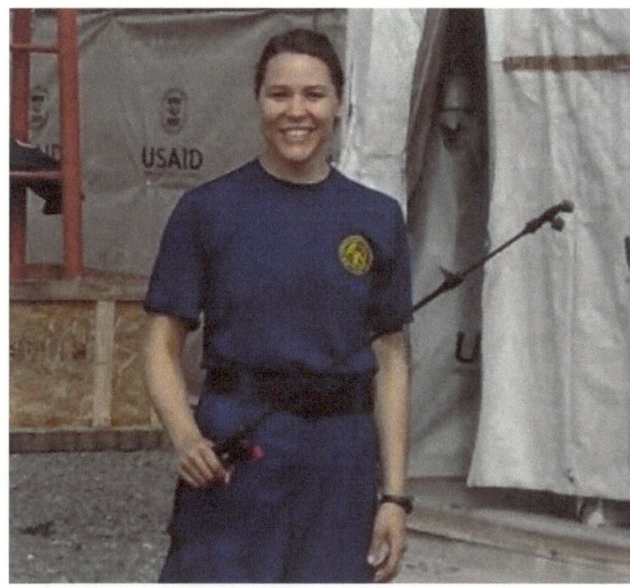

LT Freiman demonstrates the decontamination procedure of doffing.

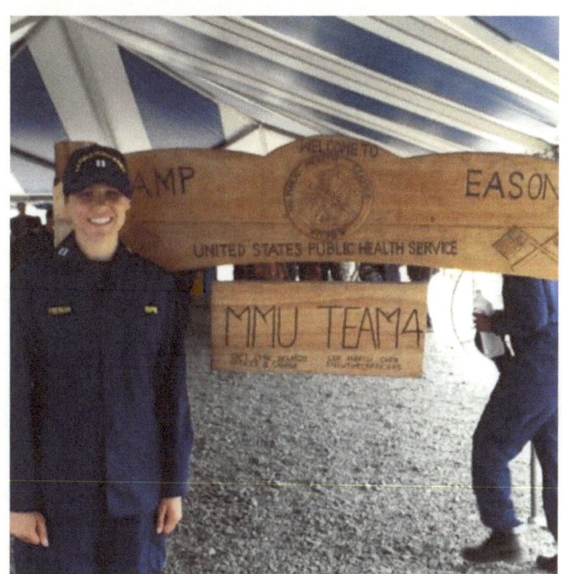

LT Freiman stands next to the homemade, wooden Camp Eason sign.

LT Anca Tabakova

"We always helped each other: building things, cooking, sharing feelings."

—Anca Tabakova, MD, MPH

LT Anca Tabakova deployed with Monrovia Medical Unit (MMU) Team 3 from January 19 to April 1, 2015. She was assigned to the administration section but spent most of her time in Liberia with the Medical Operations (MedOPS) Section. LT Tabakova's duties were mostly related to patient- and web-based Emergency Operations Center. She provided support to MedOPS from patient intake to discharge, such as preparing and maintaining the medical chart, monitoring and updating laboratory information, taking pictures, and scanning and uploading medical information. LT Tabakova spent a major part of her time transcribing the paper medical chart into an electronic WebEOC record. She created the standard operating procedure (SOP) for the Administration section's role in MedOPS. Also, LT Tabakova helped with donning and doffing and attended to other administrative requirements related mainly to personnel accountability. LT Tabakova stated, "We always helped each other: building things, cooking, sharing feelings."

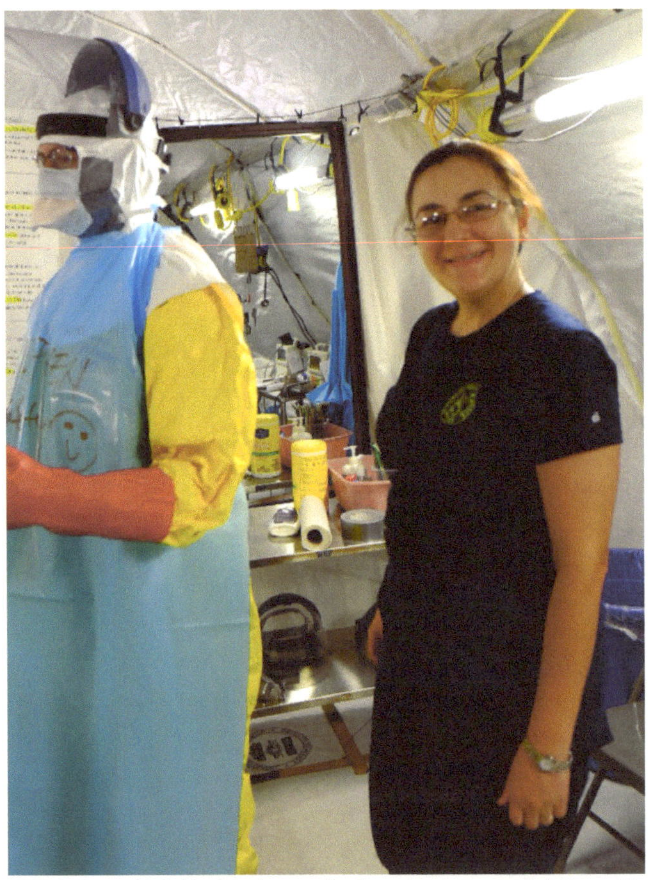

LT Tabakova *(right)* inside the medical treatment tent assisting with donning and doffing training.

LT Cody Thornton

"Do what is necessary in the moments that matter most, not for yourself but for others."

—LT Cody Thornton MPH, MBA

LT Cody Thornton's work with the West Africa Ebola outbreak started in April 2014 and extended until the end was declared in June 2016 due to his roles as manager of the US International Health Regulations program and coordinator for the US International Health Regulations IHR National Focal Point. He was responsible for ensuring the dissemination of official messages from the World Health Organization (WHO) and its Member States to the US government operation centers and key policy and response officials. He coordinated domestic and international efforts associated with Ebola preparedness and response and consolidated nationally reportable Ebola-related information to WHO and its Member States. He also served as the action officer for RADM Giberson and as the response commander for the United States Public Health Service (USPHS) Ebola Response Task Force from August to December 2014. He supported policy, logistical coordination, and administrative requirements that enabled the United States Public Health Service (USPHS) to deploy to Liberia. LT Thornton then deployed with Monrovia Medical Unit (MMU) Team 3 to Liberia as an administrative officer. As always, unforeseen needs arose, and officers stepped up to address those needs. LT Thornton says that in such times "Do what is necessary in the moments that matter most, not for yourself but for others." LT Thornton became a public information officer (PIO), drafting a number of articles and updates from the field that were disseminated to the USPHS Commissioned Corps officers, family members, the Office of the Surgeon General, the Office of the Assistant Secretary for Health, and the Office of the Assistant Secretary for Preparedness and Response (ASPR). He also supported the press conference on the Liberia-US clinical research partnership on the ZMapp Ebola treatment study held at the Liberia Ministry of Commerce and Tourism. During this event he provided guidance and de-conflicted messages for US representatives from the National Institutes of Health (NIH) and the MMU. He also served as a member of the mortuary team. In that role, he had to prepare the body of one of the MMU patients who lost his life to the Ebola virus. He also augmented the preventative medicine team in the donning and doffing duty rotation, providing relief to his teammates.

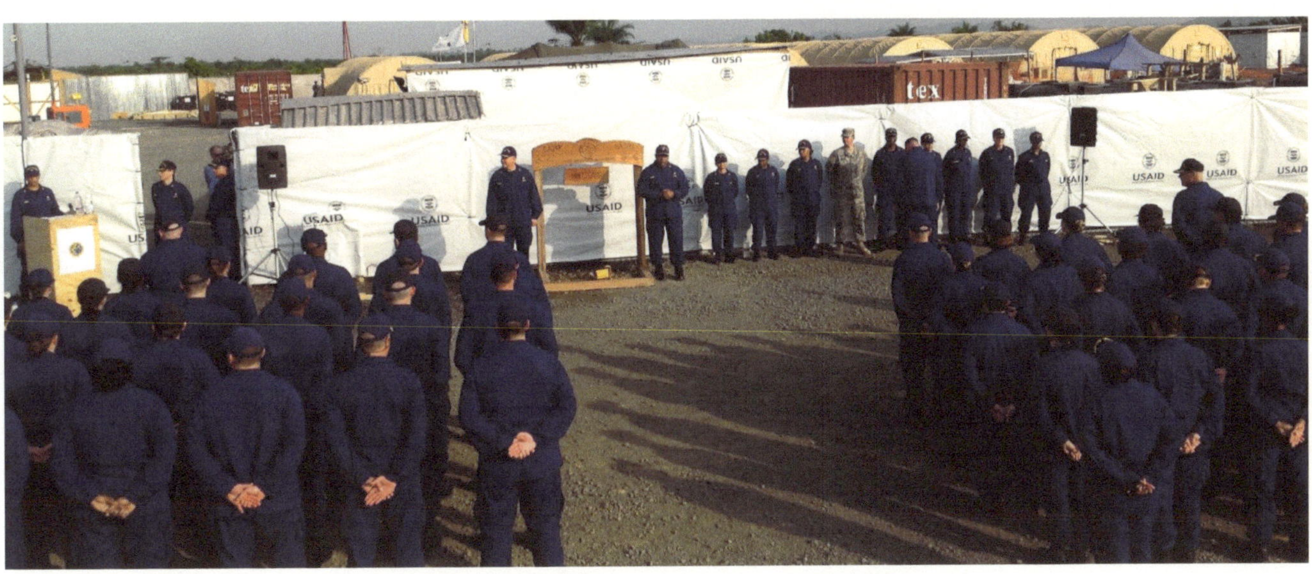

MMU Team 3 *(left)* and MMU Team 2 *(right)* in formation at the change of command ceremony.

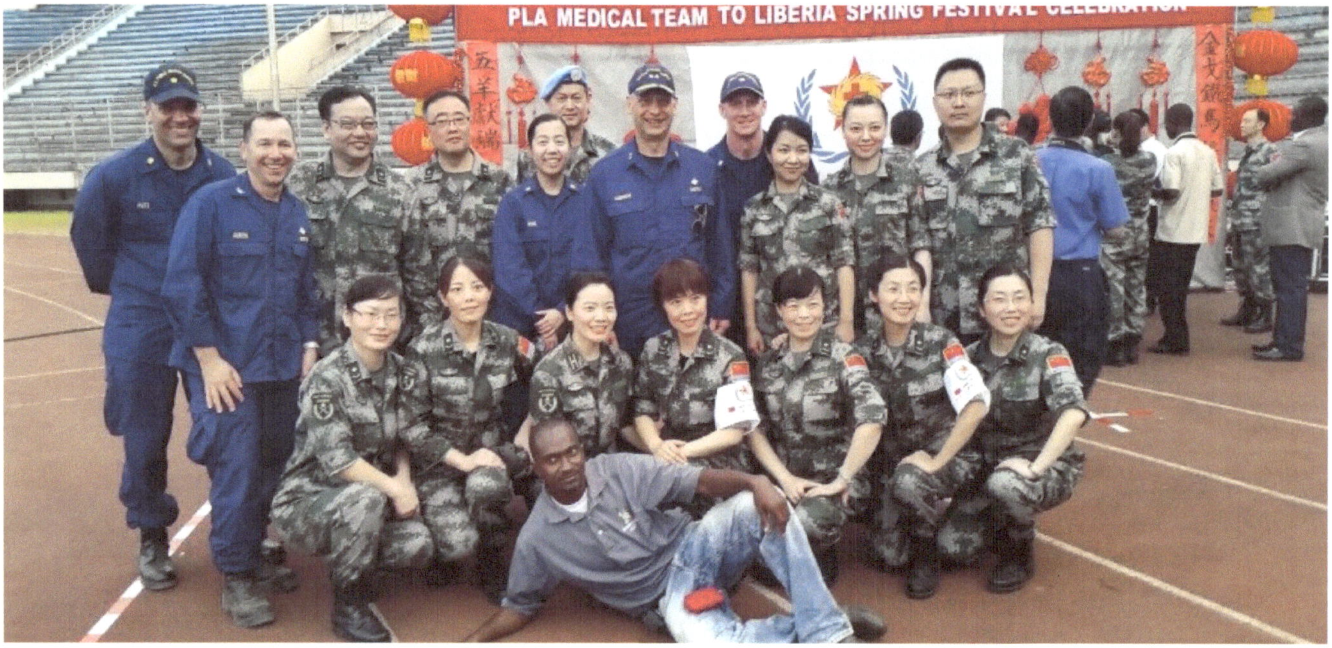

USPHS leadership and MMU representatives take a photo with Chinese Ebola Treatment Unit (ETU) leadership at a Chinese ETU–hosted Lunar New Year event.

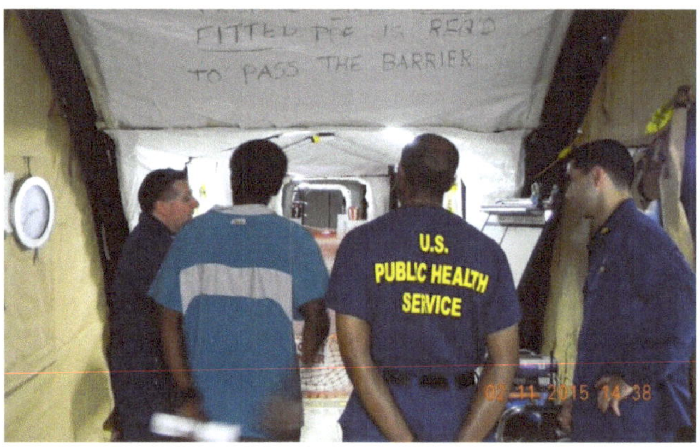

(left to right) CDR Zagame, Public Information Officer (PIO); CDR Sigh; and LT Thornton provide an explanation of the medical operations (MedOPS) and protocols to Dr. Wasambla, Director of the Tubmanberg ETU.

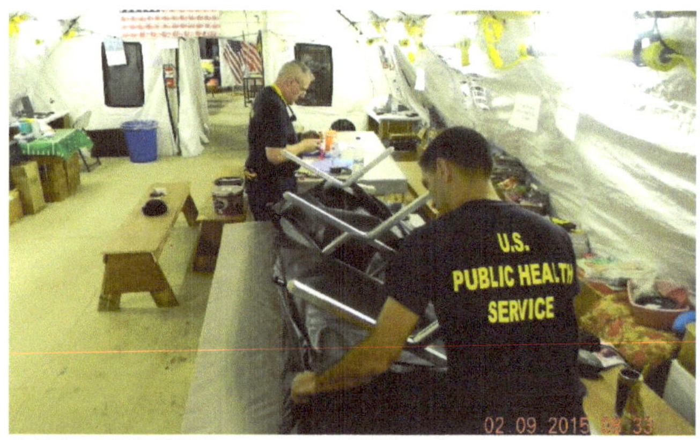

(left to right) CDR Trombley and LT Thornton fabricating mortuary team equipment from existing MMU supplies.

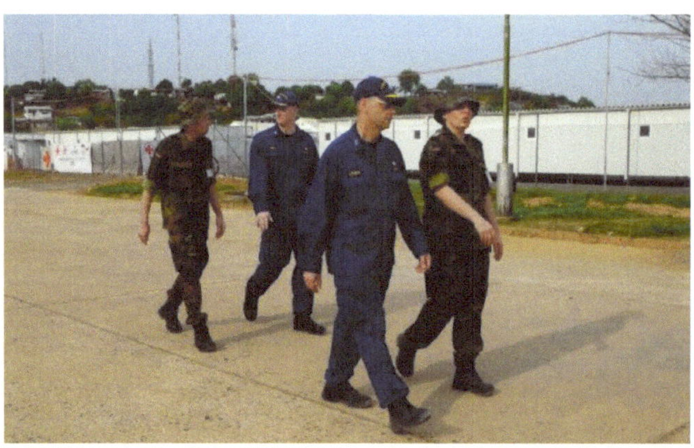

RADM Lushniak, CO of USPHS Liberia (Jan-Feb 2015), walks and talks with officers of the German Severe Infection Temporary Treatment Unit in Liberia.

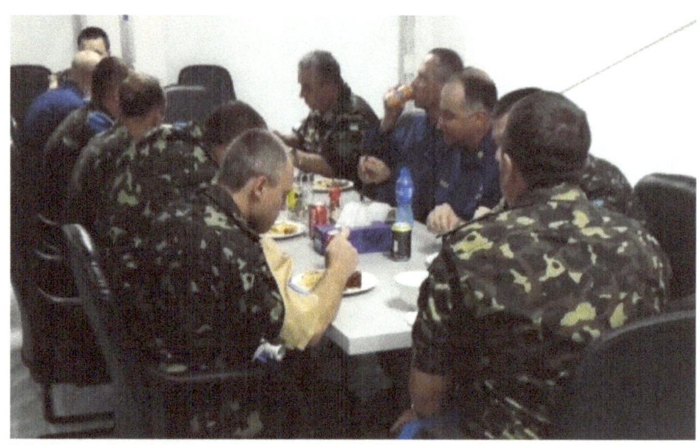

MMU leadership breaks bread with Ukrainian Detached Helicopter Unit Delegation.

LT Thornton helped strengthen team unity and boost morale in part by developing a cadence for MMU Team 3. There are a number of additional verses for different periods of the deployment, but the first and core cadence is still fondly remembered by many of the officers of MMU Team 3 and VIPs that visited the MMU during Team 3's time at Camp Eason.

Up in the morning with the Liberian sun,
Runnin' ETUs is what we call fun.
Treatin' patients, runnin' labs, and wearin' PPE:
Safety's number one, and that's how it's gotta be.
That's not all that's going on, we're only half done;
Admin, logs, and mental health ensure the mission's won.
So listen up, here's why we're here. Our mission is clear:
Steadfast treatment for our Ebola fightin' peers.
So when we come consider it done and know our service name,
"The US Public Health Service," we're winning this game.

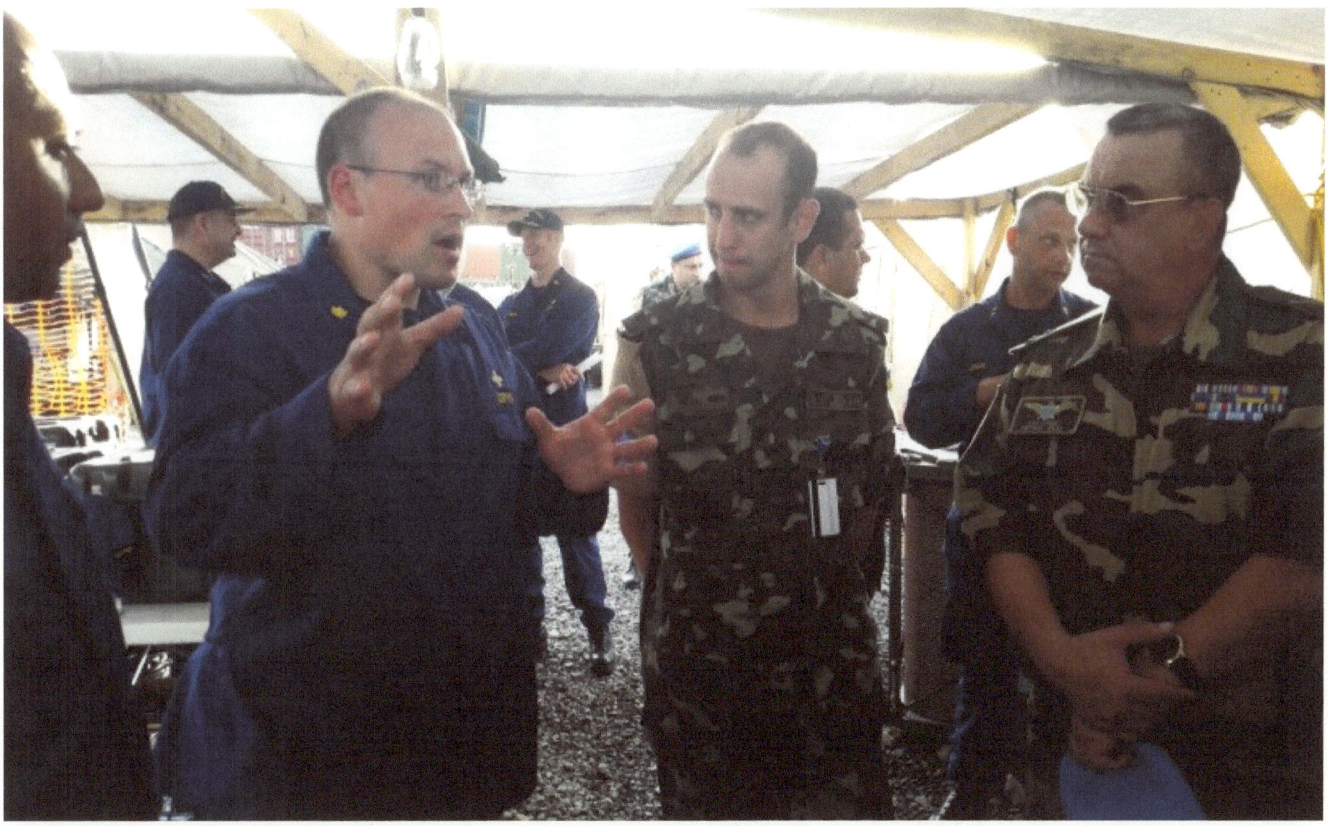

CDR Thakur, LCDR Deptola, and CDR Crump (out of frame) discuss safety considerations regarding doffing, intake, and mortuary procedures with Colonel Plis, Commanding Officer (CO) of the Ukranian Detached Helicopter Unit.

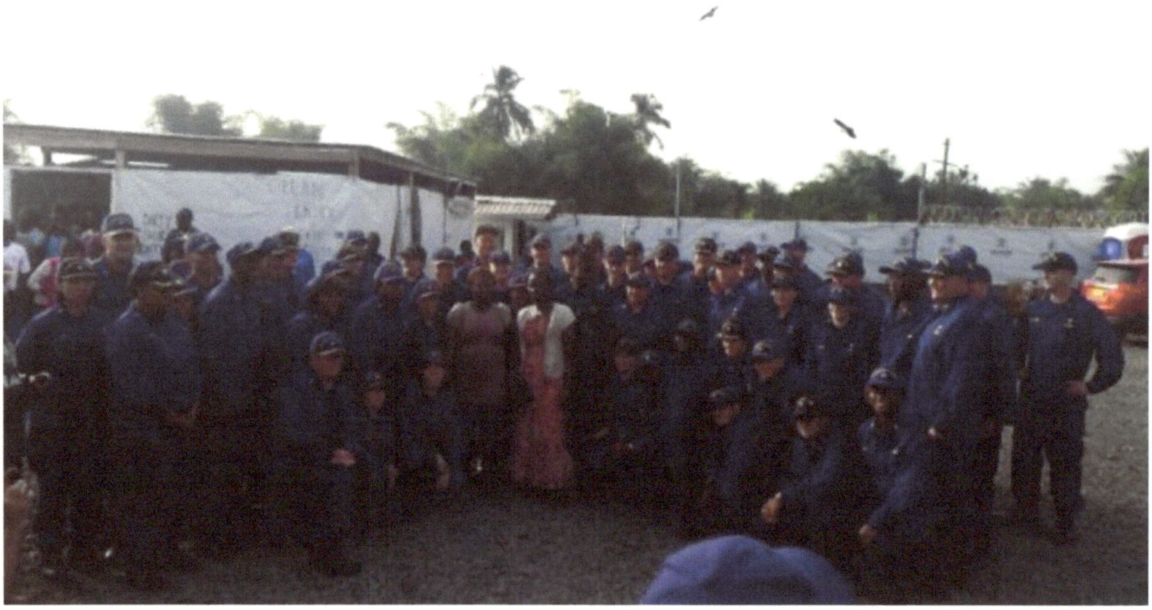

Marphen Yardola *(right)* and her sister Stephanie Yardola *(left)* pose for a picture with MMU Team 3. Marphen was the last Ebola patient released by MMU Team 3 on March 5th.

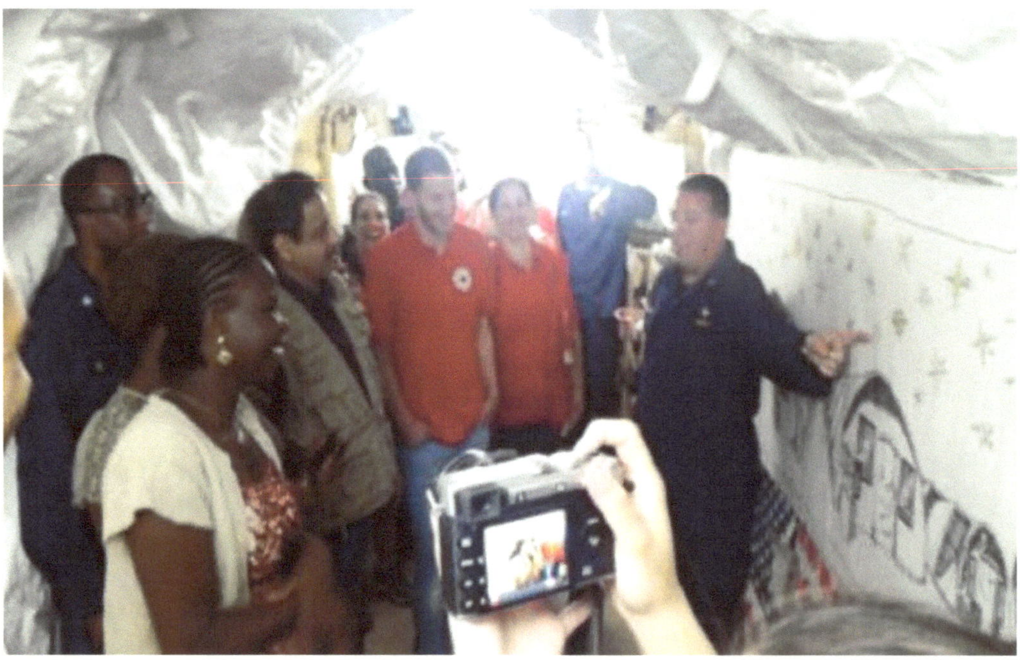

Marphen Yardola tours the MMU with CDR Zagame, MMU Team 3 Public Information Officer (PIO), and international healthcare visitors. Marphen is shown a mural that was drawn by LCDR Wong and LCDR Peng based on a photo by LT Holshue. The mural includes stars above the horizon of Camp Eason, representing all patients that have been given care through the MMU.

Thank you to the following officers who deployed as part of MMU Team 1

"First In"

Deployed from October 19 — December 20, 2014

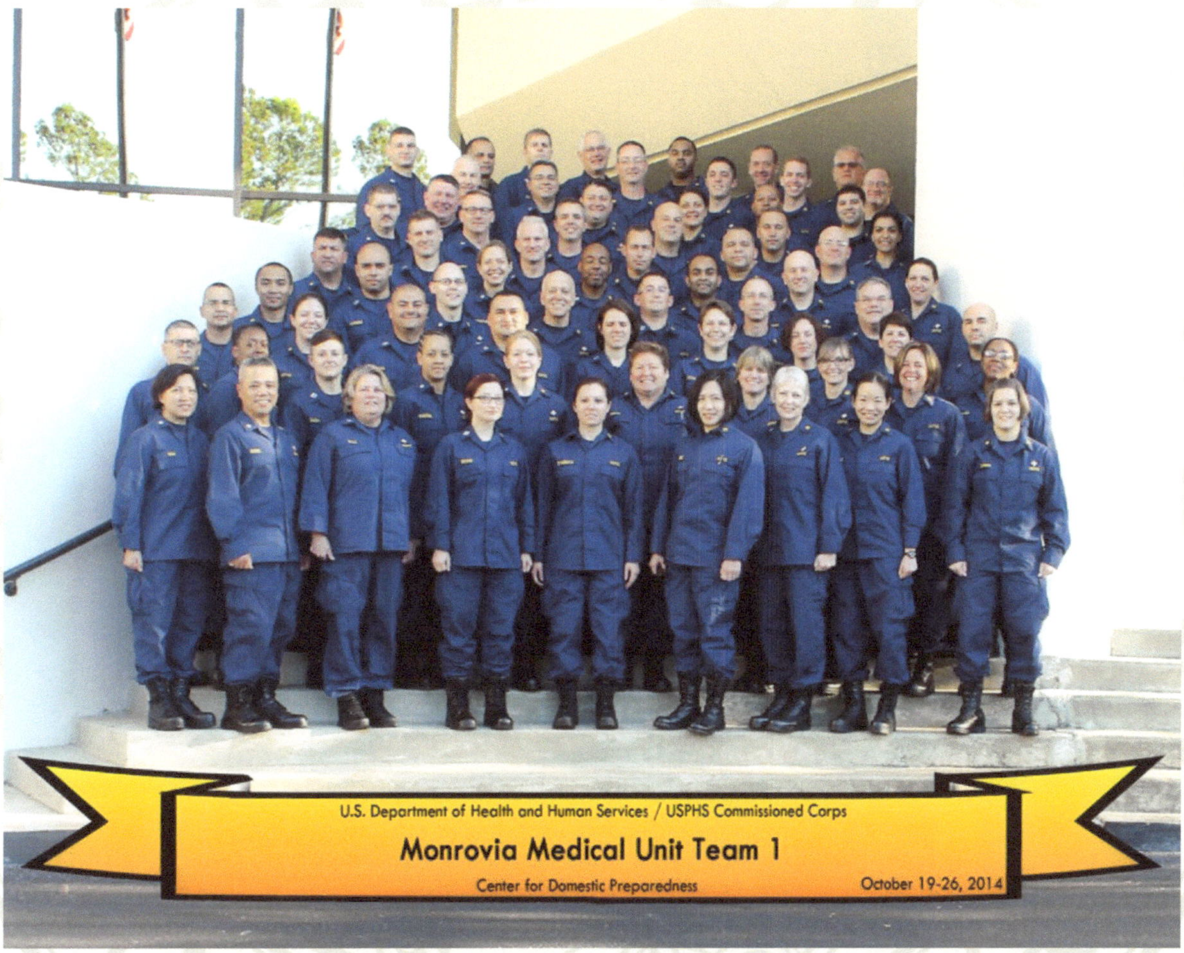

MMU Team 1

Attended CDC Ebola Training at the Center for Domestic Preparedness, Anniston, Alabama, from October 19–26, 2014

Thank you to the following officers who deployed as part of MMU Team 2

"Built on Excellence"

Deployed from December 4, 2014 — March 4, 2015

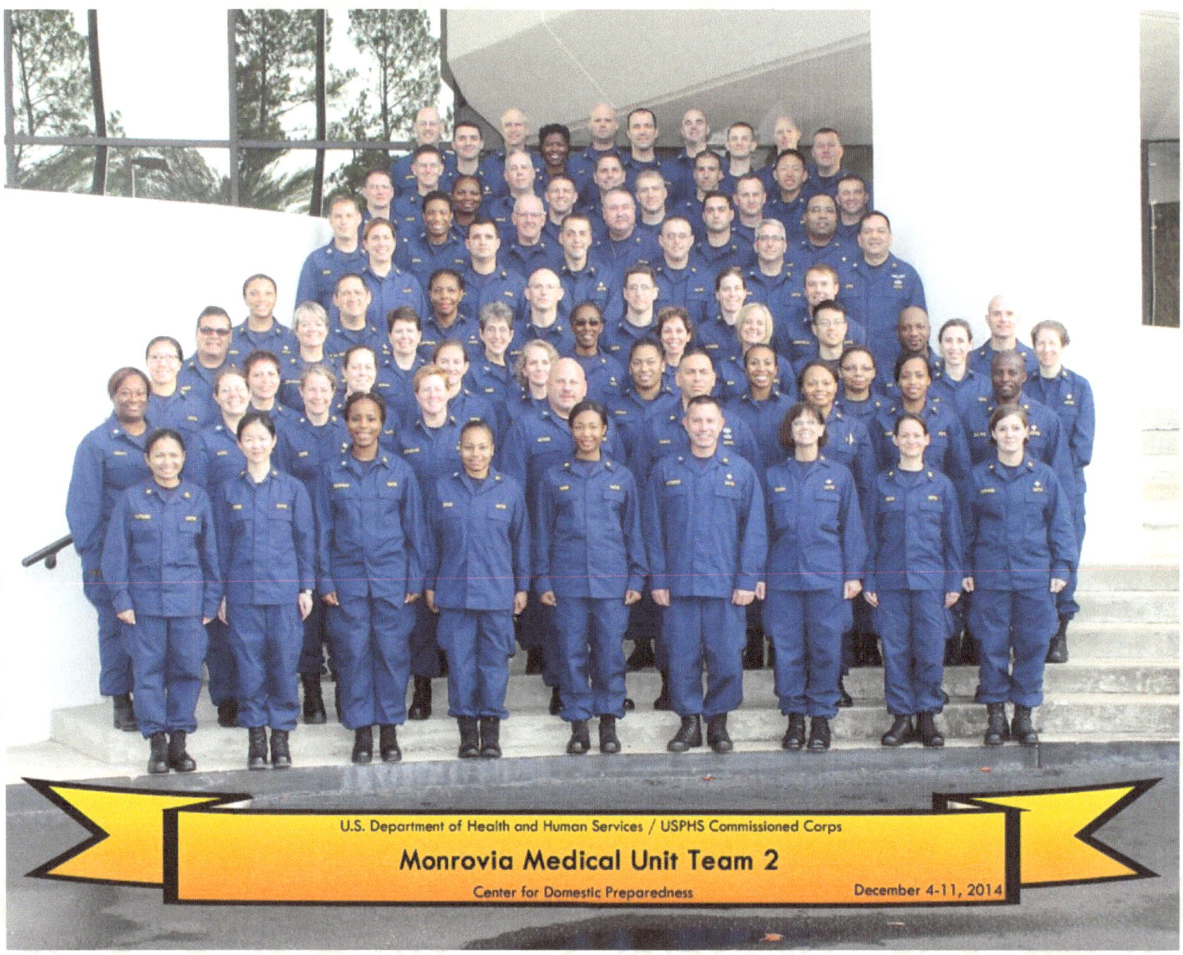

MMU Team 2

Attended CDC Ebola Training at the Center for Domestic Preparedness, Anniston, Alabama, from December 4–11, 2014

Thank you to the following officers who deployed as part of MMU Team 3

"Steadfast Treatment and Enduring Hope"

Deployed from January 20 — March 23, 2015

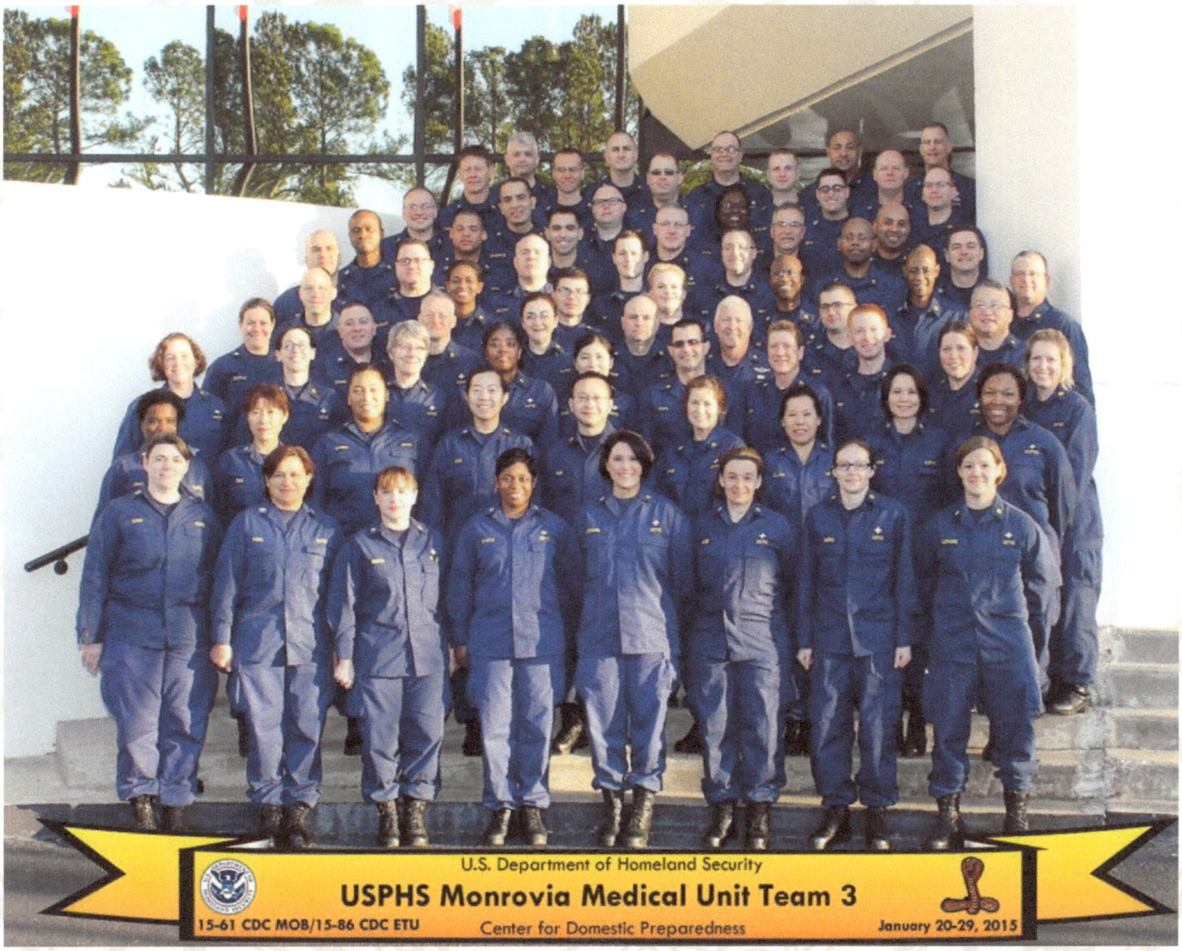

MMU Team 3

Attended CDC Ebola Training at the Center for Domestic Preparedness, Anniston, Alabama, from January 20–29, 2015

Thank you to the following officers who deployed as part of MMU Team 4

"Legacy of Hope"

Deployed from March 6 — May 21, 2015

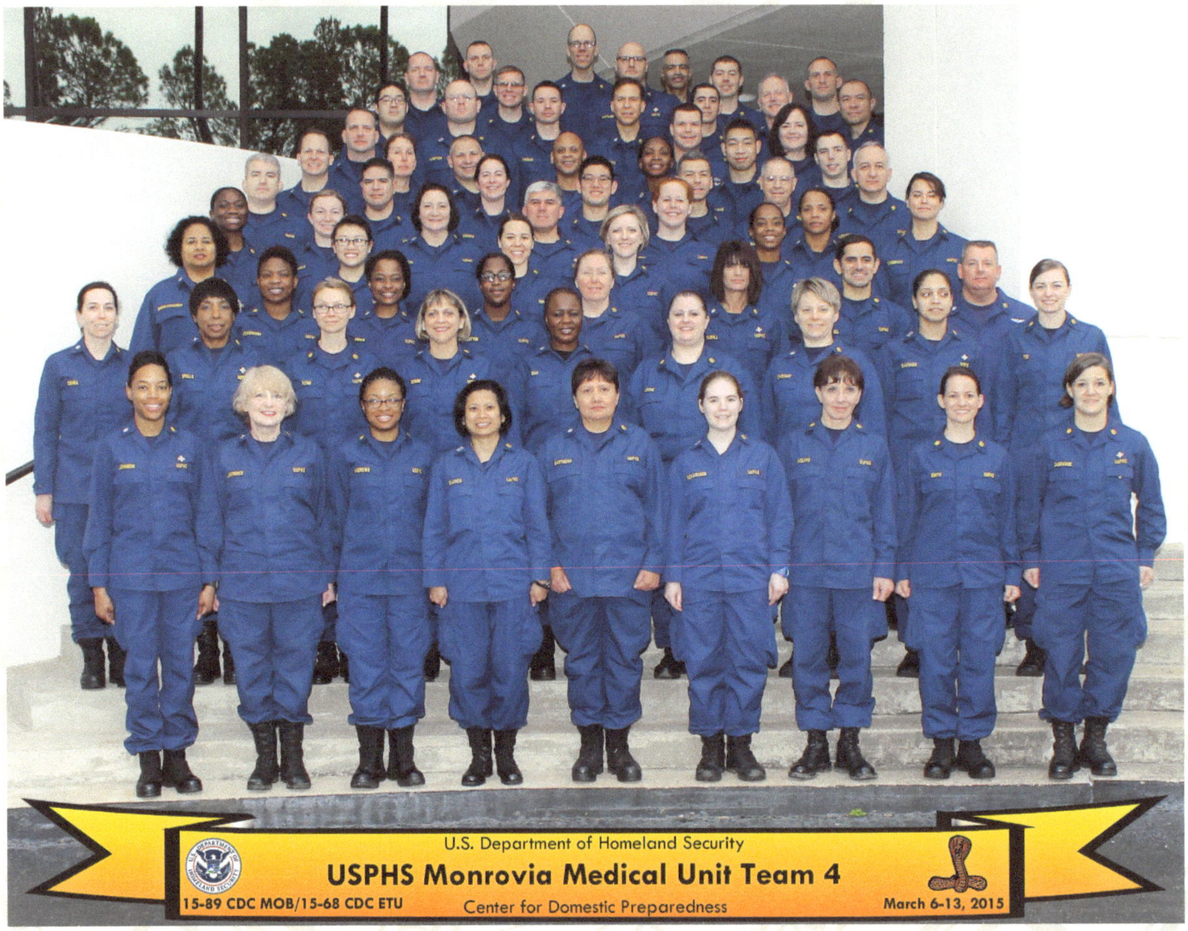

MMU Team 4

Attended CDC Ebola Training at the Center for Domestic Preparedness, Anniston, Alabama, from March 6–13, 2015

MISSION COMPLETE

Written by Julie Erb-Alvarez, MPH, CPH
CAPT, USPHS

The 2014–2016 Ebola crisis response remains unprecedented in the history of the USPHS Commissioned Corps. The Corps served in both West Africa and the US in a variety of public health and clinical roles and ultimately proved crucial in stopping the largest Ebola epidemic in history at its source. As demonstrated so eloquently in this document, Commissioned Corps health services officers served on the front lines and in direct support of operations throughout this response. These deployments collectively demonstrate the value of the Health Services category—multidisciplinary in approach—responding to fill many roles and filling needs that would otherwise go unfilled.

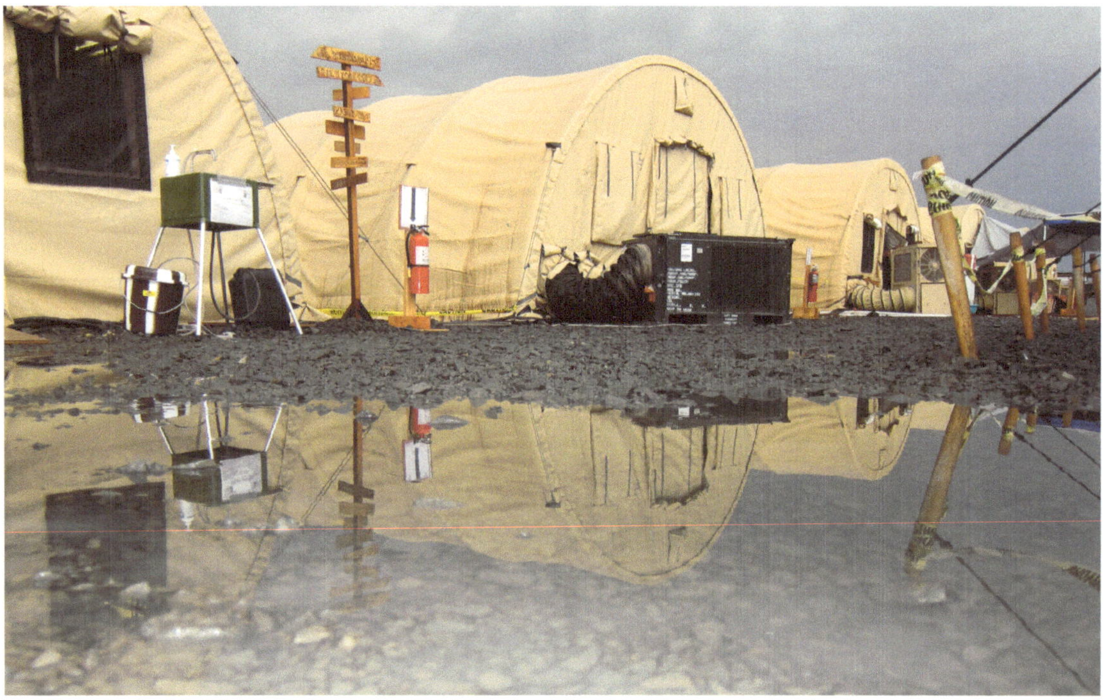

"This is truly unique to our Health Services category—to have officers with such diverse disciplines to pull from to fill such a broad range of needed deployment skillsets. The USPHS Commissioned Corps—and equally the Health Services category—stands ready to respond in future times of crisis and public health need, which are sure to come in our ever-changing world."

Presidential Unit Citation

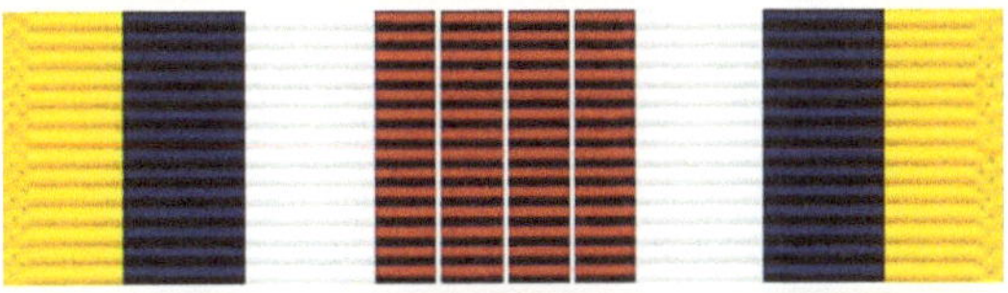

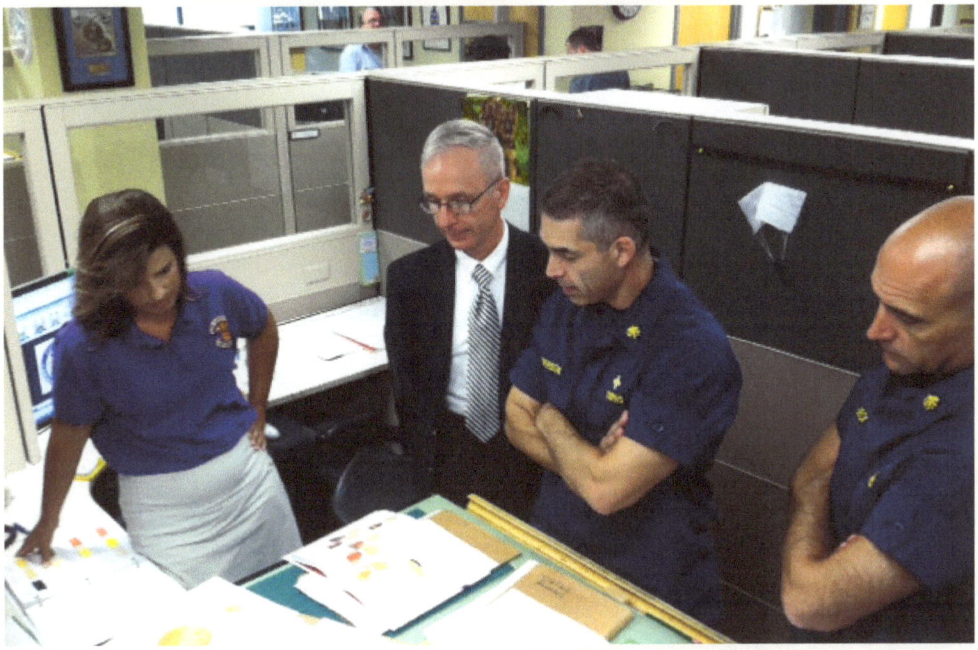

A visit to the Institute of Heraldry (TIOH) where RADM Giberson *(middle)* reviewed designs with CAPT Beck *(right)*, and TIOH staff *(left and left middle)*.

"In early December 2014, discussion commenced about how to recognize our Corps—as we envisioned this response would be successful and historic. These discussions included fact-finding and the idea for the Presidential Unit Citation (PUC) and other unique campaign awards. We engaged early with TIOH in this effort. As part of the US Army, TIOH furnishes heraldic services, such as the organization and design of decorations, flags, streamers, agency seals, coats of arms, badges, and medals, to all uniformed services and branches of the federal government. Our work with TIOH encompassed research, design, development, standardization, quality control, and other services which are fundamental to the creation and custody of official heraldic items—a necessary step in the approach to a new award."

—Assistant US Surgeon General RADM Scott Giberson

Golden Yellow	This color represents generosity and elevation of the spirit. It symbolizes our roots in quarantine medical service ("quarantine yellow") and willingness to put service before self, to protect, promote, and advance the health and safety of the nation.
Navy Blue	This color represents truth and loyalty. It symbolizes our maritime and sea service history, as well as our unwavering allegiance to the nation through our commissioning process and oath of office.
Brick Red	Brick red represents perseverance in battle and victory. It symbolizes our silent war on disease: steadfast and resolute.
Four Red Stripes	This represents our four core values exemplified in the Ebola response: leadership, service, integrity, and excellence.
White	This color represents purity, peace, sincerity, and freedom from disease. It symbolizes our diplomacy, partnerships, and outcomes with our missions both domestically and internationally.

September 23, 2015

My Fellow Officers,

Tomorrow, in an Oval Office ceremony, the President of the United States will present the first Presidential Unit Citation to the Commissioned Corps. The PUC is the highest unit-level award that can be bestowed upon a uniformed service, and I am pleased to share that President Obama will confer it to the Corps in recognition of your extraordinary courage, performance and sacrifice in the fight to contain the Ebola outbreak.

Receiving the PUC is a tremendous honor that our entire service has earned. Throughout our long and proud history, the Commissioned Corps of the U.S. Public Health Service has led on many notable public health achievements and saved countless lives by eradicating disease and responding to disasters. However, the Corps' effort to stem the Ebola outbreak is the most visible and widely recognized global health response in our history.

In this endeavor, the whole Corps was engaged. From the first set of officers sent to West Africa to track the disease and treat sick healthcare workers to those who supported the mission at domestic quarantine stations or backfilled positions within their agencies – wherever there was a need, the Corps responded. The PUC recognizes all of you for the work you did to save lives, bolster international confidence and protect the homeland.

Last Friday, I had the privilege of reuniting with our very first patient from the Monrovia Medical Unit. Alvin Davis came to visit some of the officers who took care of him while he was sick. As we talked, I couldn't help but think about the fear, doubt, and anxiety that gripped the entire world during the outbreak. At a time when so many others might have chosen to retreat, President Obama asked you to step forward. And you did.

You extended your arms in service. When our neighbors needed us the most, we responded decisively and without hesitation. You performed valiantly and exemplified the leadership, integrity and excellence that our fellow Americans – and people throughout the world – have come to expect of the Corps. In doing so, you have made all of us very proud to wear the uniform.

I say to all of you, "Bravo Zulu!" Congratulations on bringing home this incredible honor. You are truly the guardians of public health.

With pride and gratitude,

VADM Vivek H. Murthy
19th U.S. Surgeon General

Vivek Murthy

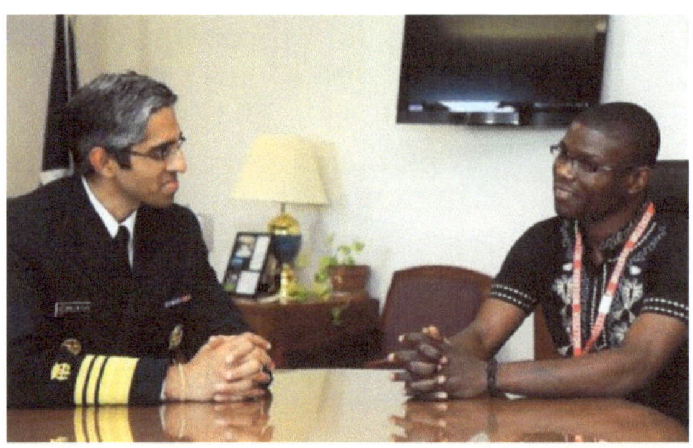

DEPARTMENT OF HEALTH & HUMAN SERVICES

Public Health Service

Office of the Surgeon General
Rockville, MD 20852

Dear Fellow Officers,

Today is perhaps a better day than most to remind you of the important role that we play as public health officers and to thank you for your continuing service to our nation. You serve our nation day after day as each of you work to "protect, promote, and advance the health and safety of our nation." You serve our nation in times of public health crisis.

Last week I had the honor of visiting with our team training in Anniston, Alabama for deployment to Liberia. I was impressed with our fellow officers -- officers enthusiastic and dedicated to the mission, proud to be part of the response, and filled with the right balance of enthusiasm and anxiety. They came as individuals and then a week later boarded a flight to Monrovia as a team-- Commissioned Corps Ebola Response Team I, USPHS Monrovia Medical Unit. They joined with our advance team led by acting Deputy Surgeon general RADM Scott Giberson and now make up a contingent of 73 officers deployed to Liberia by USPHS. Many other of our fellow officers are or have been deployed with CDC, NIH, and ASPR both stateside and in Africa. We send them all wishes to remain safe and do great things! For those not deployed or awaiting deployment, it is critical to take on the tasks of using science to educate those around us about Ebola!

On Wednesday, I had the honor of being at the White House for a special ceremony honoring those who have served or will serve in Africa. Standing behind the President were volunteers from NGO's, medical groups, and two of our own Corps officers. For the third time in the last several weeks (first at his CDC speech, then at the UN, and yesterday at the White House) , President Obama specifically mentioned the important role of the US Public Health Service in his words -- this level of mention from the President is a first in my over 26 years in uniform.

To read his remarks see here.
You can see the video here.

Before the speech, acting Assistant Secretary for Health Dr. Karen DeSalvo, CAPT Dan Beck, and I had the unexpected honor to meet the President as he walked down the hall of the West Wing. He had just been briefed on Ebola activities, stopped to greet us, and wanted us to know that the Corps was "doing a tremendous job" and that we "were already making a difference there!"

We do live in interesting times. Let us all stay prepared and be ready to further serve our nation. Thank you all for your service!

Be proud of the uniform you wear!

Sincerely,

RADM Boris D. Lushniak

Boris D. Lushniak, MD, MPH
acting US Surgeon General

1) You can read his remarks here: https://obamawhitehouse.archives.gov/the-press-office/2014/10/29/remarks-president-american-health-care-workers-fighting-ebola

2) You can watch the video here:
https://www.youtube.com/watch?v=7izW8tydtfo&feature=youtube_gdata

The President of the United States takes pleasure in presenting the PRESIDENTIAL UNIT CITATION to

PUBLIC HEALTH SERVICE COMMISSIONED CORPS

For service as set forth in the following

CITATION:

For extraordinary courage and the highest level of performance in action throughout the United States Government's response to the Ebola outbreak from Sept 9, 2014, to May 1, 2015. Upon my direction, the Commissioned Corps established and staffed the Monrovia Medical Unit to provide direct patient care, restore hope, and bolster international confidence. Commissioned Corps officers were the only United States Government asset to provide direct patient care to health care workers with Ebola in West Africa. Operations also involved highly specialized skills in epidemiology, laboratory services, and incident management. The Corps' activities helped turn the tide of the outbreak and exemplified unwavering dedication to their mission of protecting, promoting, and advancing the health and safety of the Nation. This Presidential Unit Citation awarded to all officers of the Commissioned Corps of the U.S. Public Health Service recognizes dauntless resilience and outstanding performance in the face of danger and uncertainty. The officers' tireless commitment to this response reflects great credit upon the Commissioned Corps and upholds the highest traditions of the uniformed services of the United

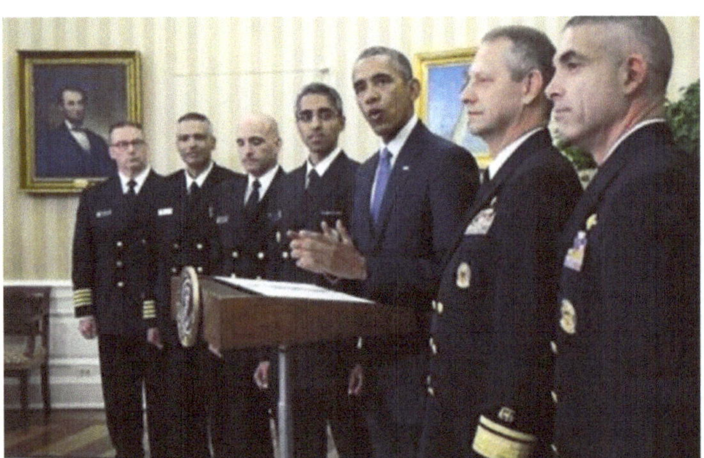

Photo by Manuel Balce Ceneta. *(left to right)* CAPT Edwards, CAPT Belardo, Health Services Officer (HSO); CAPT Beck; VADM Murthy; Commander-in-Chief President Barack Obama; RADM Lushniak; and RADM Giberson in the Oval Office during the presentation of the Presidential Unit Citation (PUC) to the USPHS Commissioned Corps.

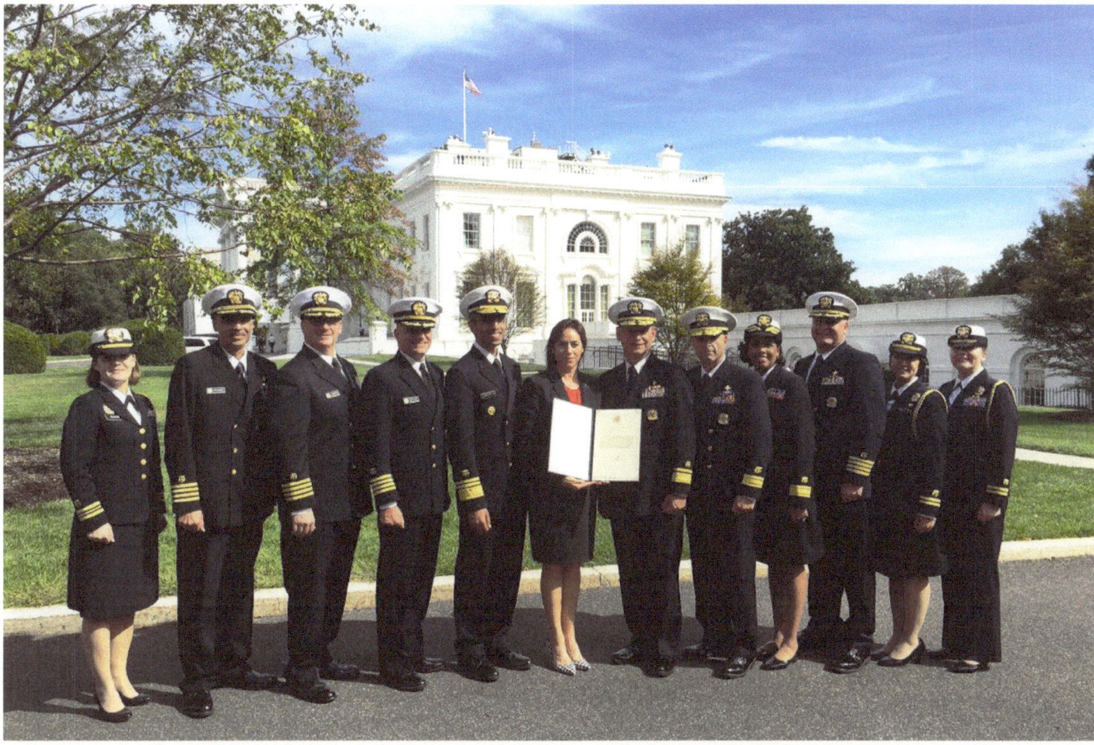

From left to right: CAPT Belardo, CAPT Edwards, CAPT Beck, US Surgeon General VADM Murthy, Acting Assistant Secretary for Health Karen DeSalvo, CAPT Lushniak, Assistant US Surgeon General RADM Giberson, RADM Trent-Adams, and CAPT Coppola after the Presidential Unit Citation (PUC) presentation in the White House.

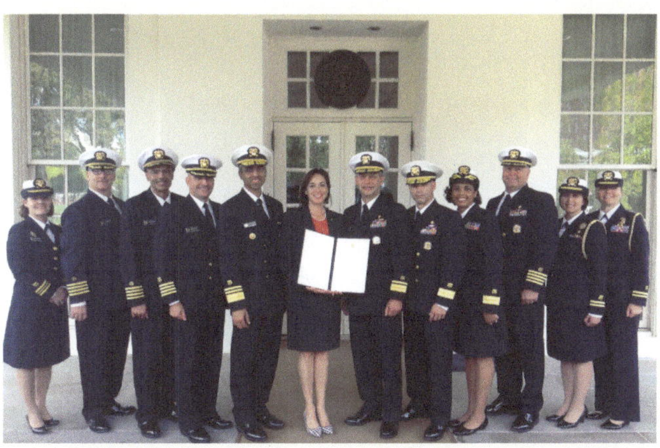

(left to right) CAPT Edwards, CAPT Belardo, CAPT Beck, US Surgeon General VADM Murthy, Acting Assistant Secretary for Health Karen DeSalvo, CAPT Lushniak, Assistant US Surgeon General RADM Giberson, RADM Trent-Adams, and CAPT Coppola after the PUC presentation in the White House.

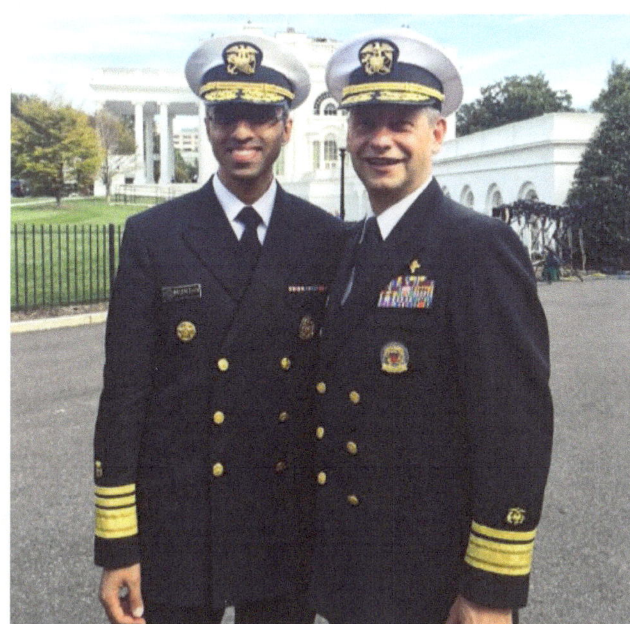

US Surgeon General Murthy and RADM Lushniak after the PUC presentation at the White House.

III

114TH CONGRESS
2D SESSION

S. RES. 540

Commending the officers of the Commissioned Corps of the Public Health Service for their work in fighting Ebola.

IN THE SENATE OF THE UNITED STATES

JULY 14, 2016

Mr. COONS (for himself and Mr. ISAKSON) submitted the following resolution; which was considered and agreed to

RESOLUTION

Commending the officers of the Commissioned Corps of the Public Health Service for their work in fighting Ebola.

Whereas the Commissioned Corps of the Public Health Service (in this preamble referred to as the "Commissioned Corps") traces its antecedents to the creation of the Marine Hospital Service in the Act entitled "An Act for the relief of sick and disabled seamen", approved July 16, 1798;

Whereas the Commissioned Corps today consists of approximately 6,700 commissioned officers who serve in 11 specialty areas;

Whereas thousands of officers of the Commissioned Corps have deployed in the aftermath of natural disasters such as Hurricanes Katrina and Rita and Superstorm Sandy;

Presidential Unit Citation Excerpt

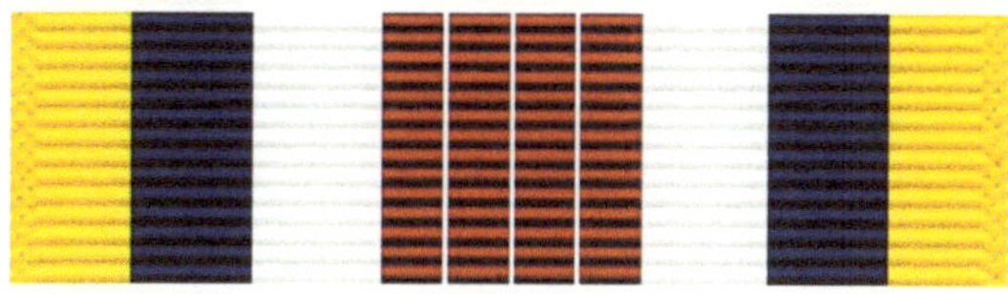

As written in the Citation, "Commissioned Corps officers were the only United States Government asset to provide direct patient care to health care workers with Ebola in West Africa."

"I have no doubt—none whatsoever—that the US Commissioned Corps of the US Public Health Service has been, is, and will remain, a critical force to preserve and protect the health of our nation."

—Assistant Secretary for Health ADM Brett Giroir's remarks at the June 2018 USPHS Scientific and Training Symposium in Dallas, Texas.

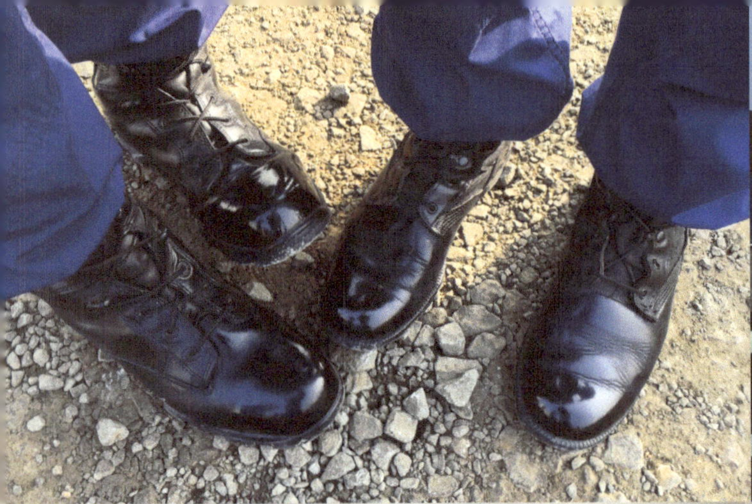

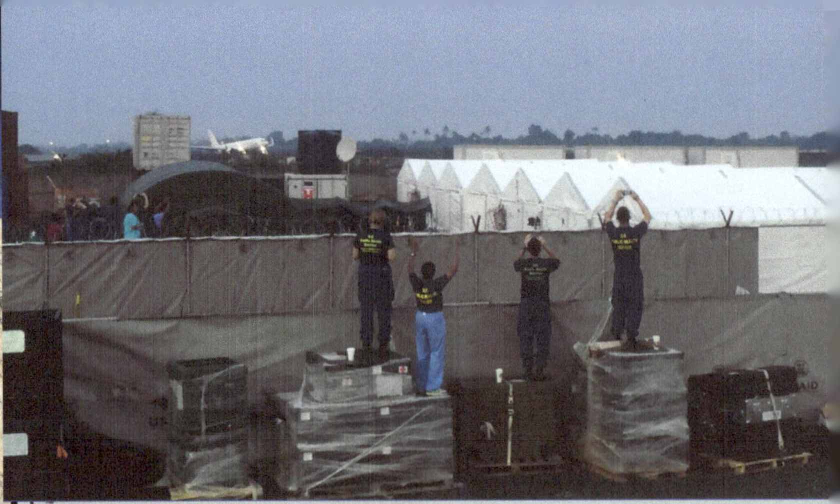

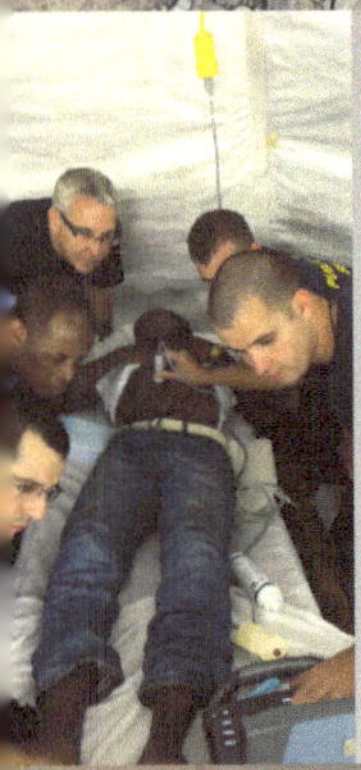

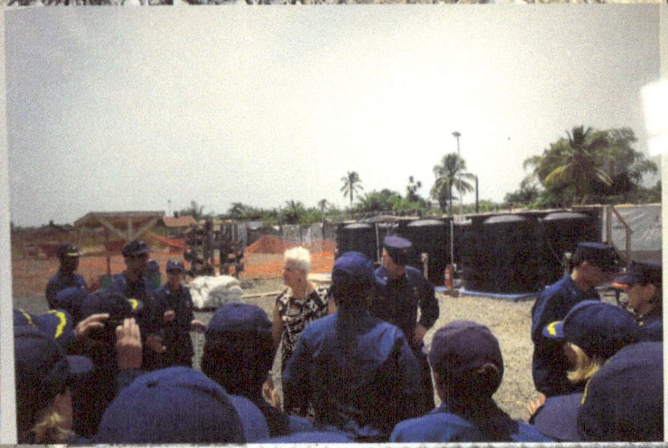

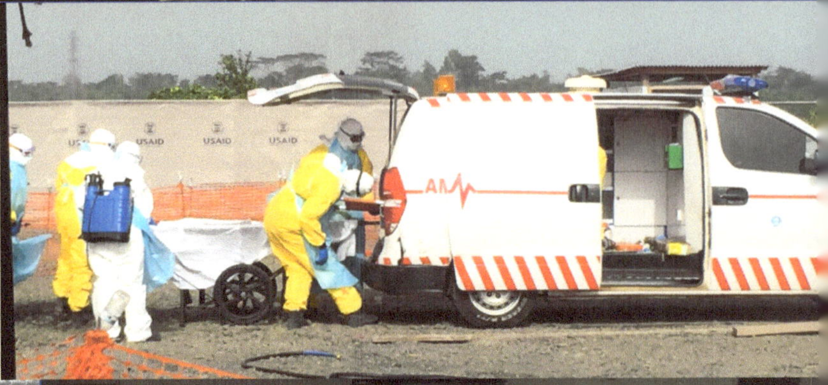
USAID

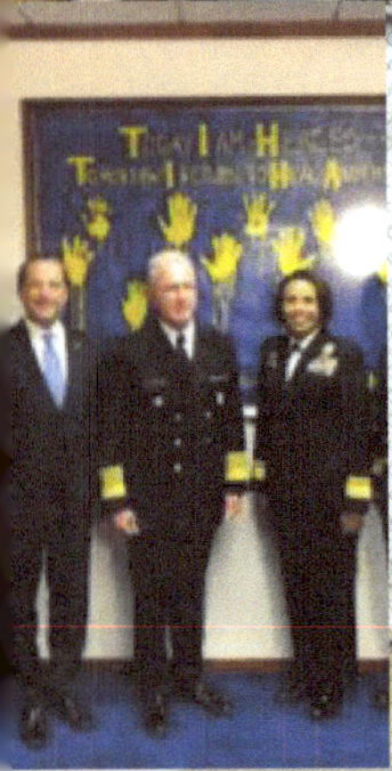

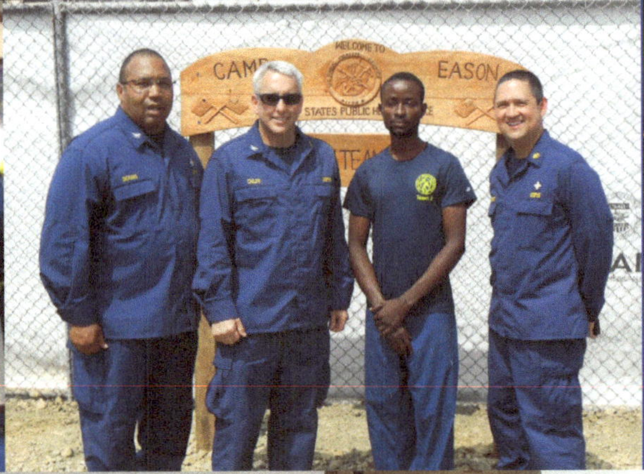
CAMP
EASON

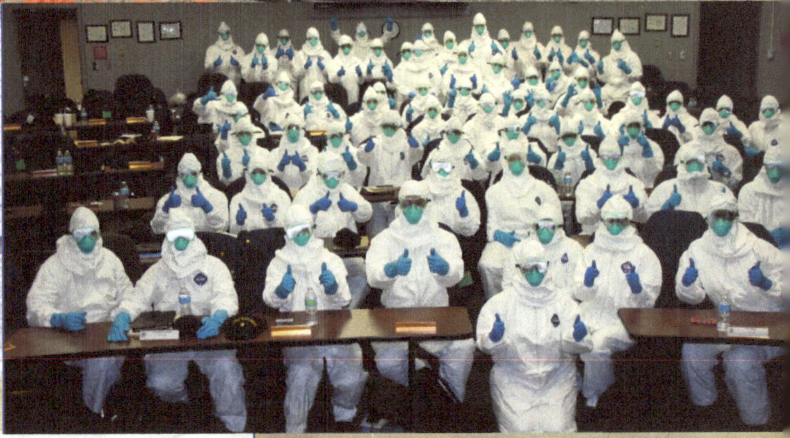

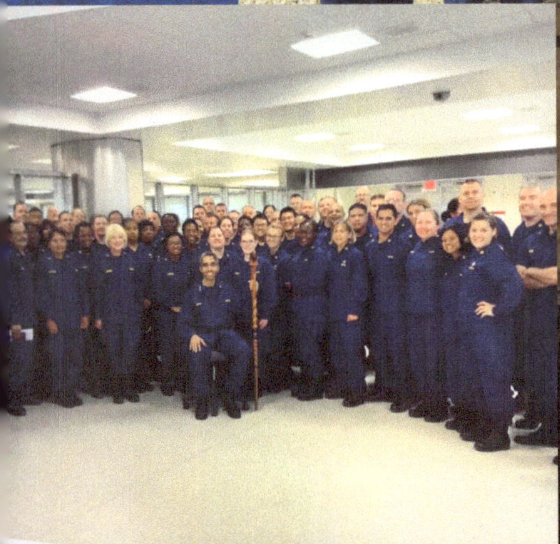

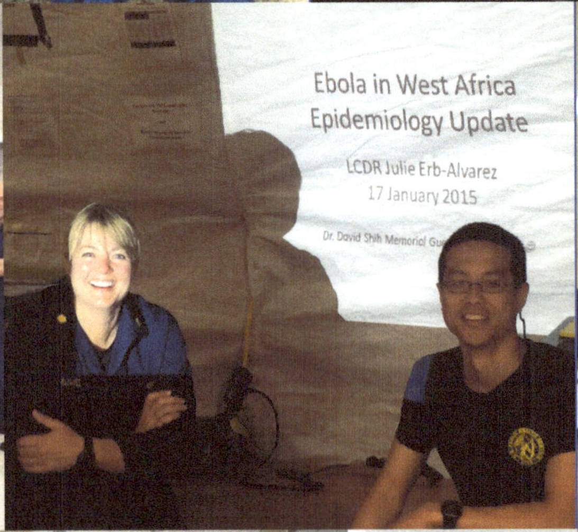
Ebola in West Africa
Epidemiology Update
LCDR Julie Erb-Alvarez
17 January 2015

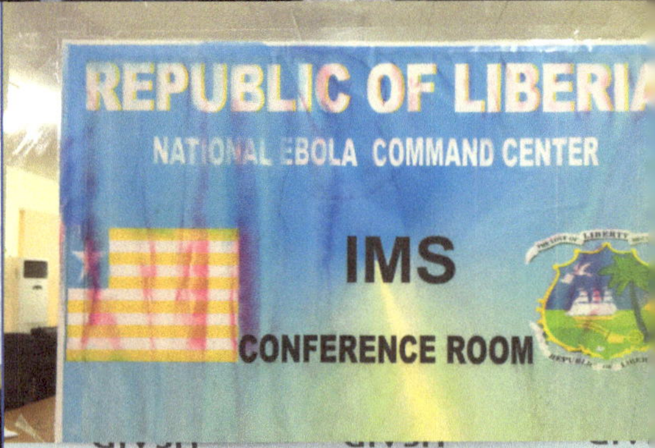
REPUBLIC OF LIBERIA
NATIONAL EBOLA COMMAND CENTER
IMS
CONFERENCE ROOM

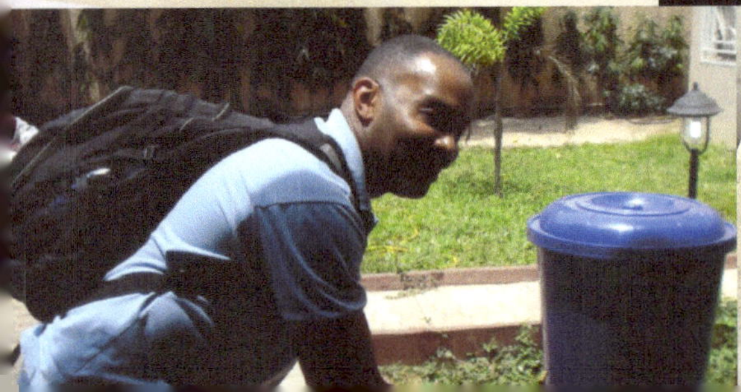

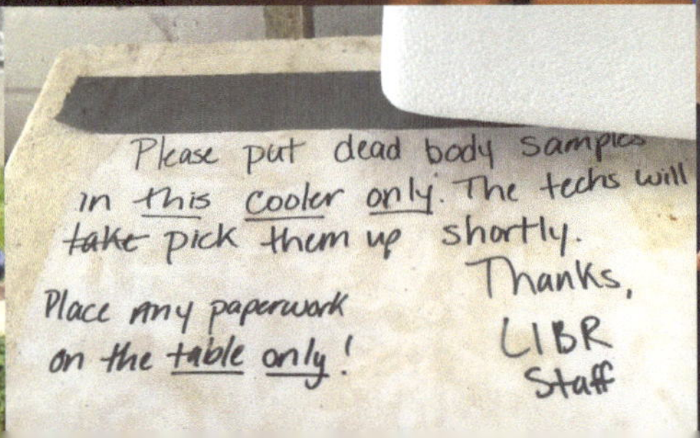
Please put dead body samples in this cooler only. The techs will ~~take~~ pick them up shortly.
Thanks,
LIBR Staff
Place any paperwork on the table only!

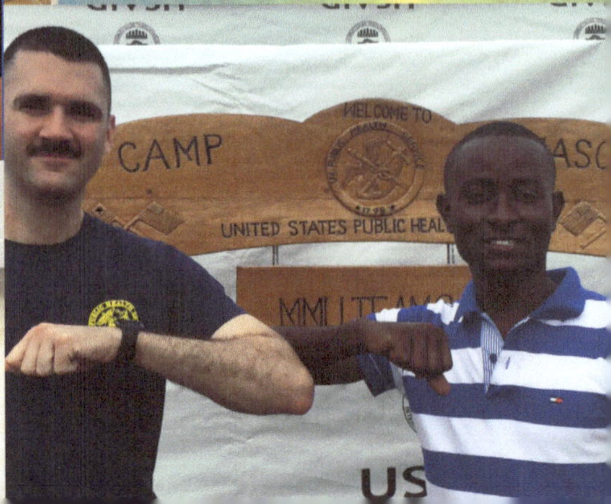
CAMP

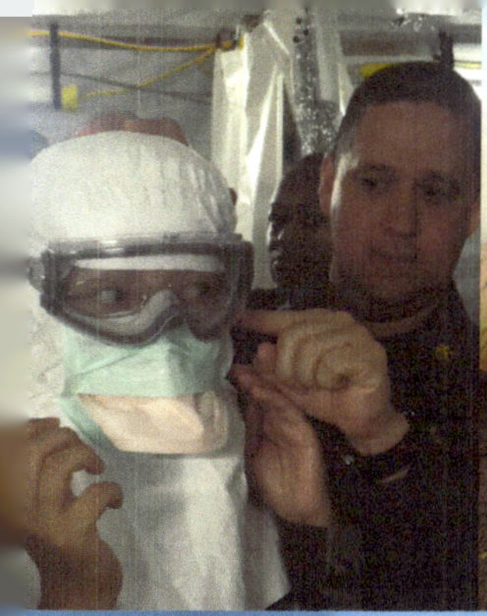

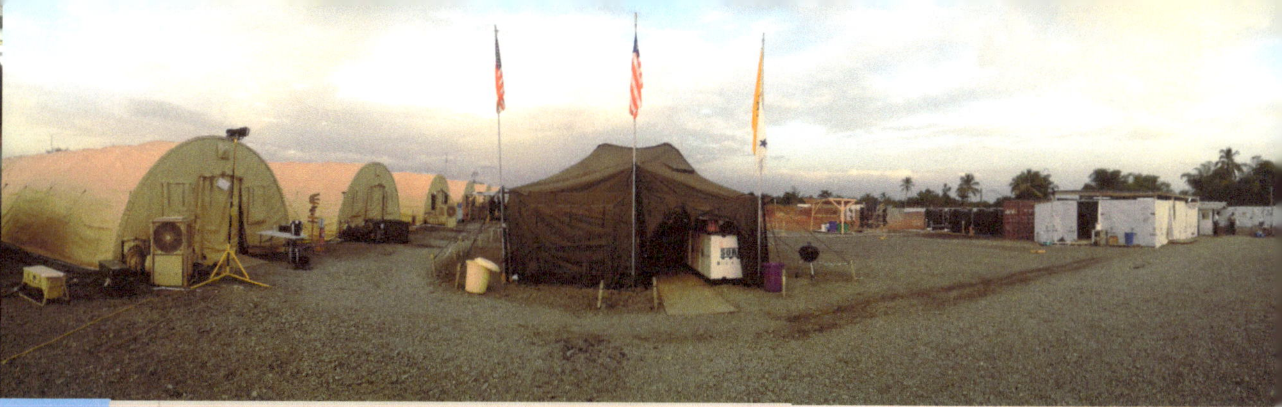

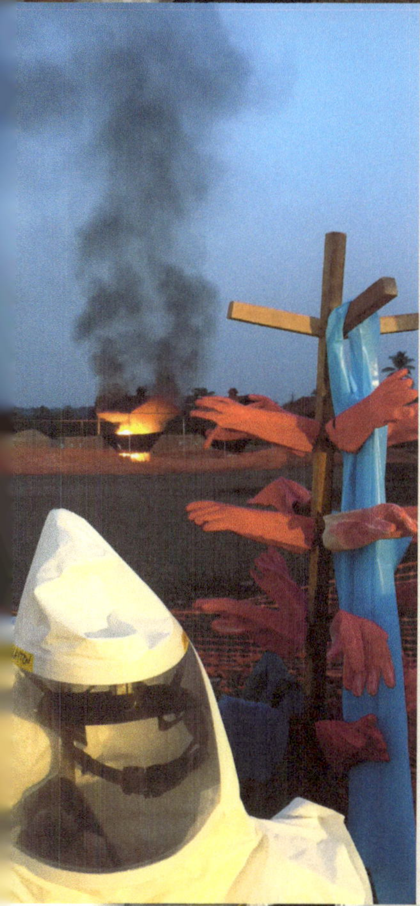

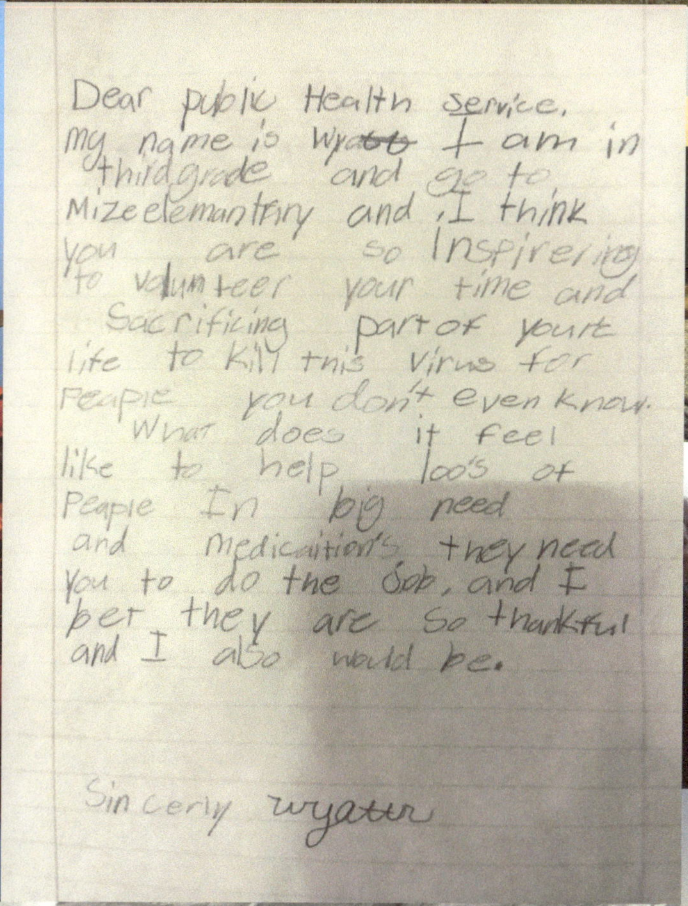

Dear public Health service,
my name is Wy~~att~~ I am in thirdgrade and go to Mizeelementary and I think you are so Inspireing to volunteer your time and Sacrificing part of youre life to kill this virus for People you don't even know. What does it feel like to help 100's of People In big need and medication's they need you to do the job, and I bet they are so thankful and I also would be.

Sincerly wyatt

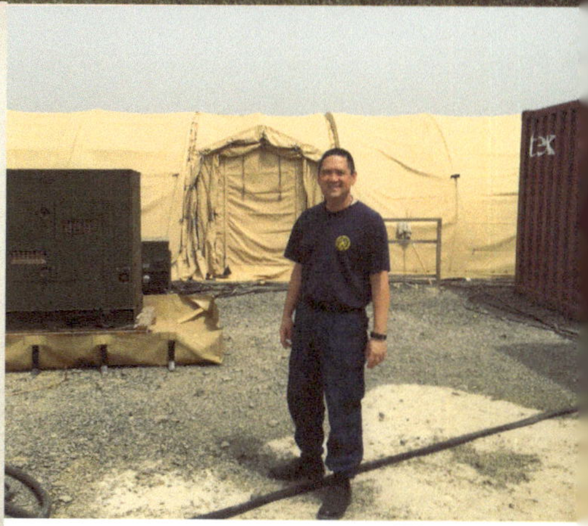

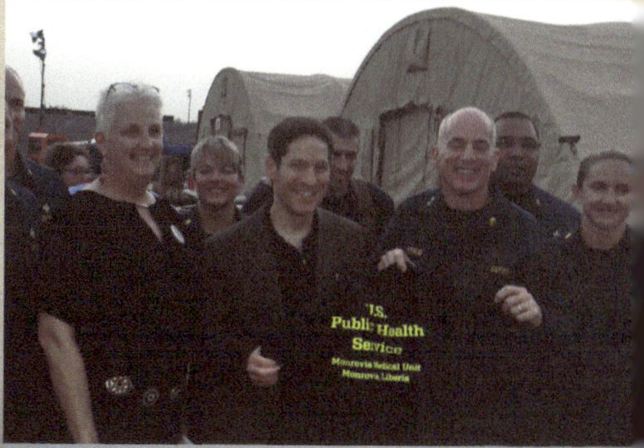

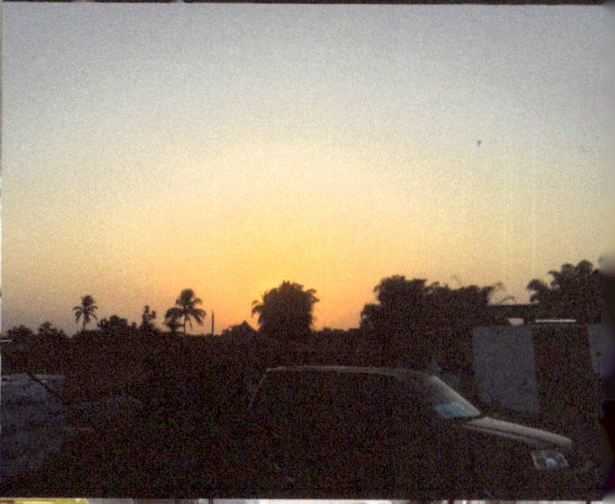

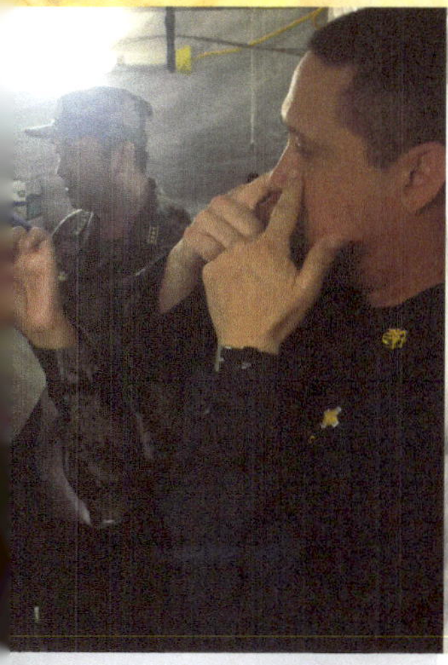

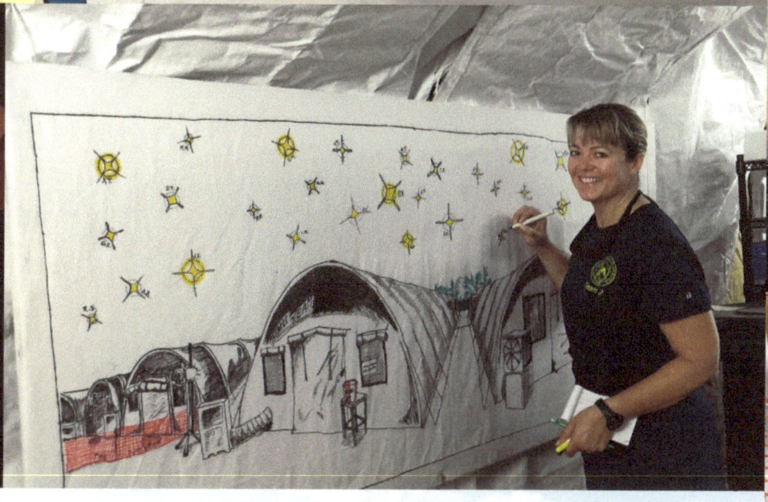

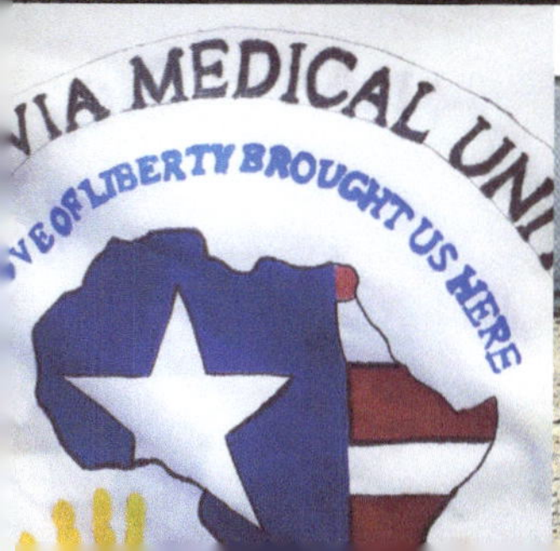

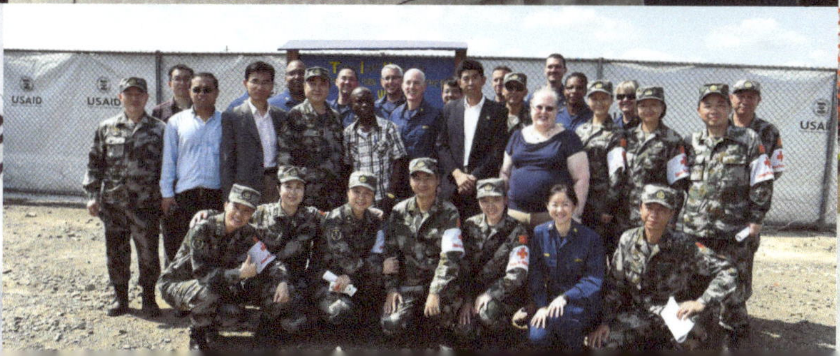

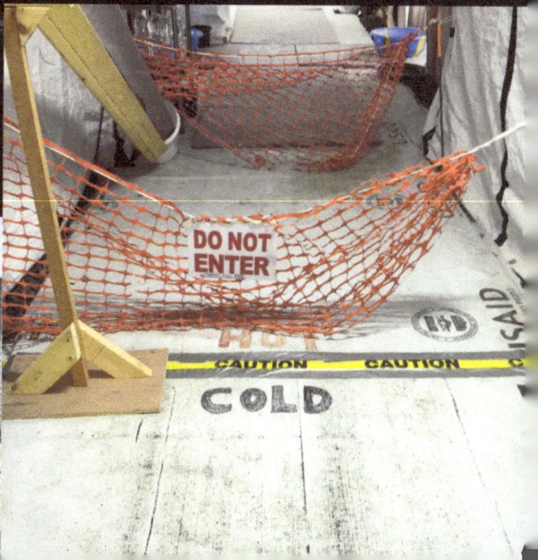

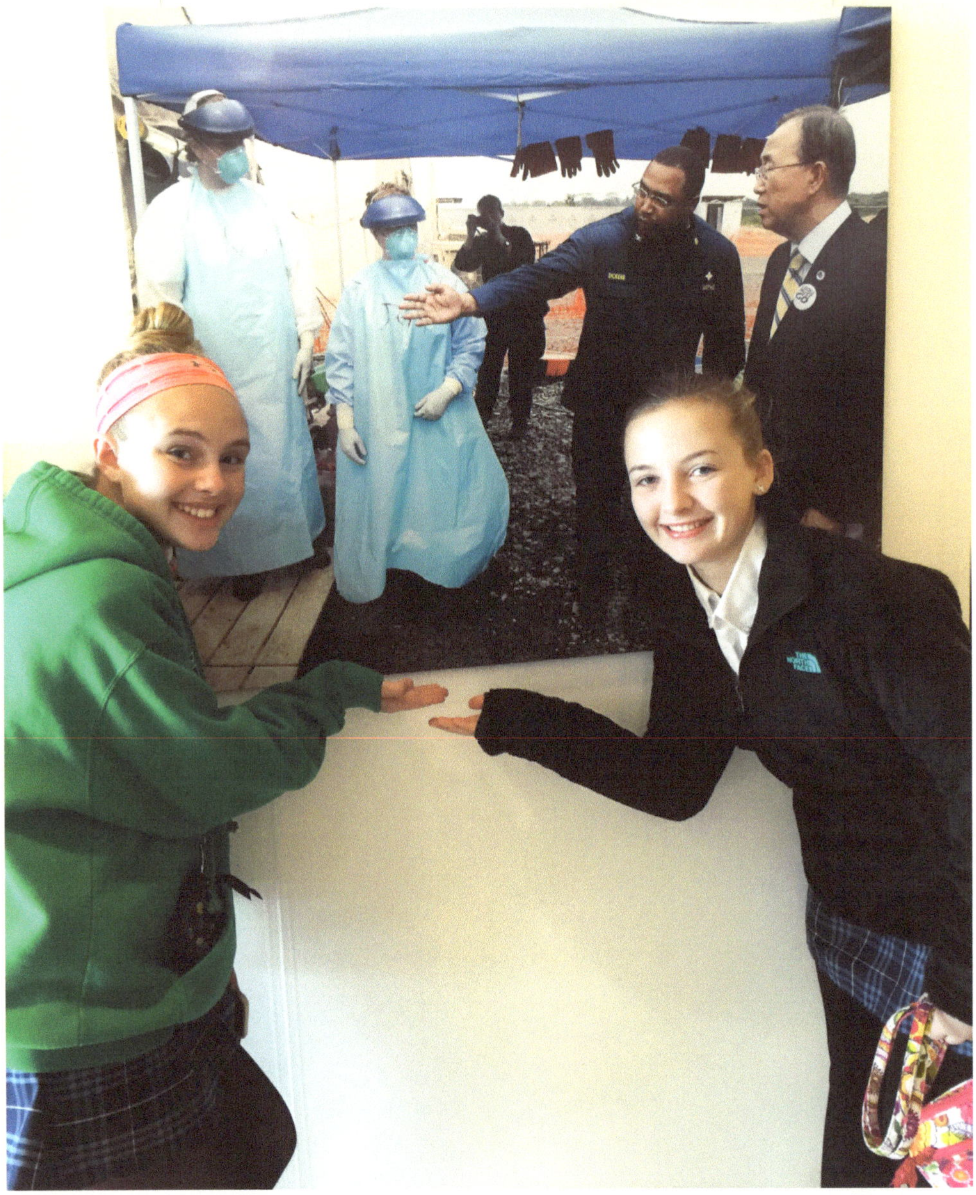

CDR Bornermann served on Monrovia Medical Unit (MMU) Team 2 *(middle, wearing personal protective equipment [PPE])*. Her niece toured the United Nations (UN) headquarters in New York City and saw this photo hanging on display. CDR Bornermann's niece texted CDR Bornermann this picture.

History of the Health Services Category

The Health Services category is the third largest category in the USPHS Commissioned Corps. The professional disciplines comprising the Health Services category provide public health leadership and service in underserved communities across the nation and throughout the world.

The traditional clinical categories were formally established in 1956, through a Federal Register Notice, to improve the promotion process for eligible officers to be considered in their discipline rather than as a single commissioned corps. Unfortunately there was no category for social and allied health services at the time. It's noteworthy to mention that in the early 1950's, two social workers were commissioned not as social workers but as "psychiatric nurses". Through a Federal Register Notice in 1959, the Health Services category was established to fulfill a critical need not only for social and allied health services but for future services that hadn't yet evolved.

Today, health services officers perform a variety of functions including direct clinical practice, program development, health planning, administration, and research. The category has grown from a small nucleus of a few officers to its present level at approximately 1,200 active duty officers. The category continues to grow and change to fulfill new health leadership roles. The Health Services motto "Multidisciplinary in Approach, Connected by Service, Advancing Public Health" attests to the wide range of skills and experience possessed by this multidisciplinary team of officers and their pride in and commitment to serving in the Commissioned Corps.

HSPAC Seal (2006–2019)[9]

"The rising yellow sun with rays represents the eternal day of our professional Public Health Service (PHS) presence anywhere in the world and our commitment to bringing light to the darkness of disease and pestilence. The blue shield signifies national service. Inside the center of the shield is a gold caduceus signifying our central role in national health, flanked on the left by a yellow lamp of learning, representing our commitment to further our knowledge and education in health. On the right is a blue lightning bolt representing our swiftness to act in protecting the public health. The white quill it crosses represents the administrative disciplines in the category and our commitment to creating national policy. The white scroll at the bottom of the shield signifies the higher ethical standard of officers and our mission. The scroll contains the words 'Strength by Diversity' which contain a wide range of skills and experience contained in the over fifty disciplines that make up the health services category."

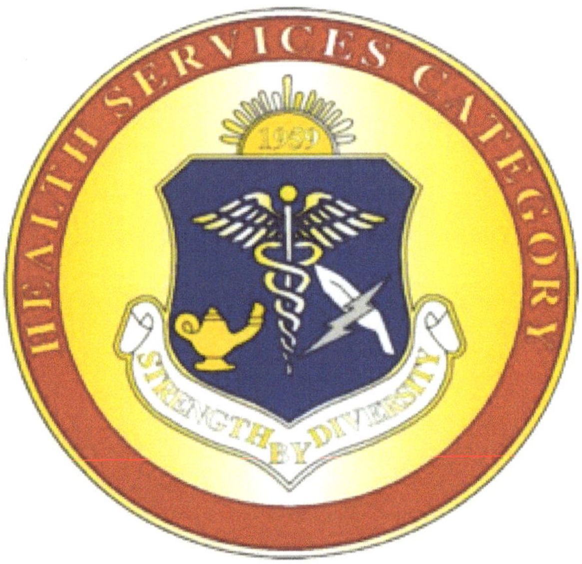

9—This version of the HSPAC seal was officially retired in 2019 and replaced with a new version. In recognition of the officers who served in the 2014-2016 Ebola response the seal under which they served is displayed here.

Acknowledgments

Health Services Category, Established 1959

Funding support provided by:

The PHS Commissioned Officers Foundation for the Advancement of Public Health (COF)

The mission of the PHS Commissioned Officers Foundation for the Advancement of Public Health is to advance public health and public health leadership for a healthier Nation. The PHS Commissioned Officers Foundation was founded on June 7, 2000 by the Board of Directors of the Commissioned Officers Association (COA). The Foundation, a not-for-profit organization, serves as the education and research affiliate of the COA. Over the past 20 years, the Foundation has matured through increased capitalization, expansion of its programmatic reach, and by assumption of new responsibilities. Their work is accomplished through five priority areas: Advocacy, Education and Training, Governance and Development, Preservation of Heritage, and Project and Research Support.

DC Branch of the Commissioned Officers Association

Thank you to the DC branch of the Commissioned Officers Association (DC COA) for providing financial l support to enable us to memorialize this historic Corps response. The mission of DC COA includes the furtherance of the mission of the Commissioned Officers Association of the U.S. Public Health Service (COA) by extending the national association's activities in the District of Columbia Metropolitan Area. In addition to cooperating in the furtherance of the mission of COA, DC COA will carry out such functions as mentoring, counseling, facilitation of discussion, and social activities on behalf of its members; fostering relations among retired, active, life, reserve, and former officers of the USPHS Commissioned Corps; protecting the rights and interests of personnel of the USPHS; and serving the community and Nation. More information can be obtained regarding DC COA at https://www.dccoa.org. Additionally, more information about the national association can be viewed at http://www.coausphs.org

New York City Branch of the Commissioned Officers Association

The mission of the Greater New York City Branch of the Commissioned Officers Association (Greater NYCOA) of the U.S. Public Health Service is to promote and protect the public health of the United States by advocating for the Commissioned Corps and its officers stationed within the Central, Northern New Jersey, and New York metropolitan area. Greater NYCOA is a vibrant, proactive, member-based local branch that supports the USPHS Commissioned Corps and its active, reserve, retired officers, and the associate families.

INDEX AND LIST

Officer Index

A

LT Allen Applegate 33
CAPT Stacey Atkins 20, 22, 23

B

CAPT Carlos Bell .... v, 13
LCDR Jennifer Bornermanniv, 94, 128
CDR Christye Brown 46
LT William Brown 46, 61, 62
CAPT Robin Hunter Buskey..... 74, 75

C

CDR Jamie Seligman 89, 90
CDR Andrew Chen 18, 85, 86
CDR Julie Chodacki 84
CDR Thomas Christl 50, 103
LCDR Jennifer Cockrill 53

D

CDR Jessica Damon .... v, 37
CAPT David de la Cruz 65, 70, 71
LCDR Sylvera Demas 32
LT Khadar Diria 60
CDR Christopher Duncan 49
CAPT Amanda Dunnick 25, 26

E

CAPT Julie Erb-Alvarez ....iv, v, 37, 102, 103, 118
CDR Idongesit Essiet-Gibson 27
CAPT Stacy Evans 38

F

CDR M. Sonsy Fermin 73, 84
LCDR Karen Forbes .... v, 65, 100
LT Jennifer Freiman 107

G

CDR Anthony Garza 88
LCDR Elizabeth Garza .... v, 54
LT Roberto Garza 59

H

LCDR Mouhamed Halwani v
CDR Leslie Hausman 29
LCDR David Hunter 55, 74
LCDR Arthur Hurst 33

J

LCDR Matthew Johns ....ii, iv, 79, 98
LT Jennifer Johnson 34
CDR Joseph Roth Jr. 80
LT Heather Joseph 72, 76, 80

K

CDR Ibrahim Kamara 28
CDR Debra King 51
CDR Erich Kleinschmidt 87

L

LCDR Philip Lafleur 99
CDR David Lau 91, 92
LCDR Meredith Pyle 56
LT Jennifer Johnson 34, 105
CDR Carolina Luna-Pinto 30

M

CAPT Robin MacGowan 72
CDR Charlene Majersky 81
LCDR Kate Migliaccio ..... v, 16, 19, 95
CDR Kenneth Monahan 79
LT Samantha H. Morgan 35
CAPT Rendi Murphree 43
CDR Ericka Murray 52

O

LCDR Osamede Onaghise 57, 58

P

CDR Tracy Pace 93
LCDR Skip Payne 97
LT Taran Pierce 63
LCDR Chris Poulson 96
LCDR Meredith Pyle 56

R

LT Janesia Robbs 36
CDR Joseph Roth Jr. 80
CDR Tobey Manns Royal 83

S

CAPT Michael Schmoyer 19, 78
LCDR Evelyn Seel 104
CDR Jamie Seligman 89
CAPT Angela K. Shen 44, 69
CDR Erica J. Sison 31
CDR Jacinta Smith 47, 48
CDR Torris Smith 82
CAPT Cynthia Spells 73
CAPT (Ret.) Dorothy Stephens 76

T

LT Anca Tabakova 108
LT Cody Thornton 109, 110, 111
LCDR Tracy Tilghman 104
LT Tracy Tilghman 104
LCDR Rafael Torres-Cruz 101

W

CAPT Craig Wilkins 20, 24
LCDR Lorraine Williams 106
CAPT Robert Windom 77

Acronym List

ADVON	Advanced Echelon
AFRICOM*	US African Command
APD	Anticipate, Plan, and Deter
ASPR	Office of the Assistant Secretary for Preparedness and Response
AU	African Union
BARDA	Biomedical Advanced Research and Development
BHOG	Behavioral Health Operations Group
BHW	Bureau of Health Workforce
BOP	Federal Bureau of Prisons
BSL	Biosafety Level
CAPT*	Captain
CARE	Check and Report Ebola
CBP	Customs and Border Protection
CDC	Centers for Disease Control and Prevention
CDP	Center for Domestic Preparedness
CDR	Commander
CHES	Certified Health Education Specialist
CMS	Centers for Medicare and Medicaid Services
CPH	Certified in Public Health
CO	Commanding Officer
COAST	Consolidated Overseas Accountability Support Toolbox
CONOPS	Continuity of Operations
CPO	Chief Professional Officer
CSTLTS	Center for State, Tribal, Local, and Territorial Support
CSU	Cultural Services Unit
DART	Disaster Assistance Response Team
DGMQ	Division of Global Migration and Quarantine
DHCFS	Division of Health Careers and Financial Support
DMAT	Disaster Medical Assistance Team
DNAC	Direction Nationale de l'Aviation Civile
DOD	Department of Defense
DOIC	Deputy Officer-in-Charge
EEES	Ebola Enhanced Entry Screening
EIND	Emergency Investigational New Drug
EMED	Expeditionary Medical Support
ETC	Ebola Treatment Center
ETU	Ebola Treatment Unit
EUA	Emergency Use Authorization

EVD	**Ebola virus disease**
FDA	**Food and Drug Administration**
FPO	**Field Project Officer**
FSN	**Family Support Network**
HHS	**Health and Human Services**
HPP	**Hospital Preparedness Program**
HRSA	**Health Resources and Services Administration**
HSO	**Health Services Officer**
HSPAC	**Health Services Professional Advisory Committee**
IHR	**International Health Regulations**
IHS	**Indian Health Service**
IMS	**Incident Management System**
IPC	**Infection Prevention and Control**
ISDR	**Integrated Disease Surveillance and Response**
JFK	**John F. Kennedy**
KAP	**Knowledge, Attitudes and Practice**
LCDR*	**Lieutenant Commander**
LT	**Lieutenant**
MCM	**Medical Countermeasures**
MedOPS	**Medical Operations**
MMU	**Monrovia Medical Unit**
MOH	**Ministry of Health**
MOHS	**Ministry of Health and Sanitation**
MOT	**Ministry of Transportation**
MOU	**Memorandum of Understanding**
MPH*	**Master of Public Health**
MRC	**Medical Reserve Corps**
MSF	**Médecins Sans Frontières**
MSW*	**Master of Social Work**
NETEC	**National Ebola Training and Education Center**
NGO	**Non-Governmental Organization**
NIAID	**National Institute of Allergy and Infectious Diseases**
NIH	**National Institutes of Health**
O2C2	**Office of Management and Budget Clearance Center**
OFDA	**Office of Foreign Disaster Assistance**
OGA	**Office of Global Affairs**
OIC	**Officer-in-Charge**
OMB	**Office of Management and Budget**
OMHHE	**Office of Minority Health and Health Equity**
OS*	**Office of the Secretary**
OSSI	**Office of Security and Strategic Information**
PAC	**Professional Advisory Category**

PET	Office of Pandemics and Emerging Threats
PHA*	Public Health Advisor
PHS	Public Health Service
PHU	Public Health Units
PIO	Public Information Officer
PPE	Personal Protective Equipment
PREVAIL	Partnership for Research on Ebola Virus in Liberia
PsySTART	Psychological Simple Triage and Rapid Treatment
PUC	Presidential Unit Citation
QBHSB	Quarantine and Border Health Services Branch
RADM*	Rear Admiral
RedDOG	Readiness and Deployment Operations Group
REP	Rapid Ebola Preparedness
Ret.	Retired
RING	Recognize, Isolate, Notify, Give Support
RITE	Rapid Isolation and Treatment of Ebola
RRT	Rapid Response Team
RS	Reintegration Specialist
SAMHSA	Substance Abuse and Mental Health Services Association
SAT	Services Access Team
SITTU	Severe Infection Temporary Treatment Unit
SOC	Secretary's Operation Center
SOP	Standard Operating Procedure
STRIVE	Sierra Leone Trial to Introduce a Vaccine against Ebola
TTX	Table Top Exercise
UN	United Nations
UNICEF	United Nations Children's Fund
US*	United States
USAID	United States Agency for International Development
USG	United State Government
USMC	US Marine Corps
USPHS	United States Public Health Service
Web-EOC	Web-based Emergency Operations Center
WHO	World Health Organization

*No definition appears in text

www.ingramcontent.com/pod-product-compliance
Ingram Content Group UK Ltd.
Pitfield, Milton Keynes, MK11 3LW, UK
UKHW061032310726
14089UKWH00009B/205